Dr. Ana has been a friend of mine and a colleague for several years. She is truly a pioneer in everything she undertakes with orthodontics. This book is borne out of that same spirit. Dr. Ana, thank you for taking the time to write this and for your generosity. It's a step closer to changing the world a smile at a time!

Dr. Vandana Katyal
Specialist Orthodontist, Clean, Clear, & Correct Smiles
Sydney, Australia

Dr. Ana Castilla is an amazing orthodontist and a better human being. She is the embodiment of the "American Dream" overcoming many childhood challenges. She has evolved to be a shining star in orthodontics and now feels, as her true generous nature calls, to give back and change people's lives with this book. That is so much more than just straightening teeth.

Dr. Francisco J. Garcia
Garcia Orthodontics
Miami, Florida

I have had the pleasure of knowing Dr. Ana Castilla since 2002, when The Ohio State University Dental School assigned her as my "Big" to introduce me to the dental school and show me around. Since that time, I have always known Ana to be generous, an excellent teacher, and a great ambassador for orthodontics. A really unique thing about Ana is her previous background in engineering, which established an exceptional knowledge for biomechanics—which governs tooth movement. She has become a recognized expert in our field and I am proud to have her as my colleague.

Dr. Jeffrey M. Shirck
Shirck Orthodontics
Columbus, Ohio

I have known Dr. Ana Castilla for the past few years. She is very committed to the field of orthodontics and changing people's smiles. This book will help any reader to be one step closer to the smile of their dreams. She generously shares her wealth of knowledge, her own orthodontic journey, and tips to make your smile top notch. It is a privilege to learn from Dr. Ana. My best wishes and cheers to your new smile!

Dr. Hardik Kapadia
Smile Brite Orthodontics
Dallas, Texas

I met Dr. Ana Castilla in 2011 during our orthodontic residency program at OHSU in Portland, Oregon. Dr. Castilla and I became friends and it has been an honor to be her colleague. She has become a wonderful orthodontist and business owner for whom I have the utmost respect and admiration. Dr. Castilla is a board-certified orthodontist who provides the best orthodontic care available. Not only is she a fabulous orthodontist, but she pours her heart and soul into her patients and her practice. She is the most driven individual that I know and works tirelessly to benefit her patients and her practice. Dr. Castilla believes in constant development and innovation. Whether it be attending courses to become a "Master" Invisalign provider, seeking out new advances and efficiencies in the field of orthodontics, or simply thinking outside of the box to better her patients and her practice, you will not find an individual more dedicated to providing the best care and experience. She is truly a role model not only for me, but for anyone who knows her.

Dr. Megan E. Miller
Central Ohio Orthodontics
Lancaster, Ohio

The
SMILE
of your LIFE

ANA CASTILLA, DDS, MS

The SMILE *of your* LIFE

Everything

YOU NEED TO KNOW FOR YOUR
ORTHODONTIC JOURNEY

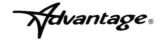

Published by Advantage, Charleston, South Carolina.
Member of Advantage Media Group.

ADVANTAGE is a registered trademark, and the Advantage colophon is a trademark of Advantage Media Group, Inc.

Printed in the United States of America.

10 9 8 7 6 5 4 3 2 1

ISBN: 978-1-64225-040-4
LCCN: 2018956861

Cover and layout design by Melanie Cloth.
Cover photography by Diana V Photos.

This publication is designed to provide accurate and authoritative information in regard to the subject matter covered. It is sold with the understanding that the publisher is not engaged in rendering legal, accounting, or other professional services. If legal advice or other expert assistance is required, the services of a competent professional person should be sought.

Advantage Media Group is proud to be a part of the Tree Neutral® program. Tree Neutral offsets the number of trees consumed in the production and printing of this book by taking proactive steps such as planting trees in direct proportion to the number of trees used to print books. To learn more about Tree Neutral, please visit **www.treeneutral.com**.

Advantage Media Group is a publisher of business, self-improvement, and professional development books and online learning. We help entrepreneurs, business leaders, and professionals share their Stories, Passion, and Knowledge to help others Learn & Grow. Do you have a manuscript or book idea that you would like us to consider for publishing? Please visit **advantagefamily.com** or call **1.866.775.1696**.

*To my mother, Geoconda, who taught me the meaning of
"whatever it takes" and helped make me the person I am today.*

Table of Contents

Introduction

It may sound cheesy, and I definitely feel like everybody says this, but writing this book was truly a labor of love for me. As those that know me well can attest, I have a very busy schedule. In fact, I think it sometimes borders on the insane. Therefore, to write this book, I gave up many weekends, sometimes working late into the night. But here's the thing. I loved every minute of it. Not because I love braces (though they are pretty cool) or because I thought there was no information on orthodontic treatment out there—there is (although maybe not all good). I loved it because it allowed me to take what I love best to the next level: connecting with others.

That is in fact one of my favorite things about my job. As an orthodontist, I get to connect with hundreds of patients and see many of them undergo a metamorphosis of sorts that is truly inspiring. Thus, my patients inspire me—as does the power of a smile. In return, I hope that in sharing my personal smile story and in providing you a guide to orthodontic treatment, I can inspire you to feel confident in taking that step and giving yourself or your loved ones the gift of a smile—the smile of your life.

Orthodontics changed my life immensely, probably more than it changes the life of the average person. But make no mistake, even if your life is not changed as much as mine, the confidence you get from a beautiful smile is priceless and worth every minute of the entire journey.

Chapter 1

MY SMILE JOURNEY

*"They say time changes things, but you actually
have to change them yourself."*
Andy Warhol

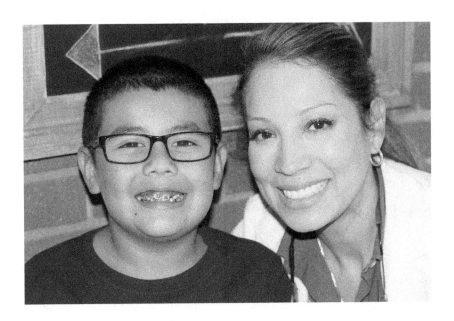

When I was a little kid, I didn't know I was poor. I mean, I knew we weren't like the families I saw on TV. I used to watch *The Brady Bunch*, and I knew the apartment I was growing up in was nothing like the house the Bradys had. And we didn't have live-in help, either. In fact, our apartment in Brooklyn was about nine hundred square feet and had two bedrooms to accommodate my family of six. So yes, I watched TV and I knew we weren't rich. What I didn't know was that being poor was something I didn't want to be. I didn't understand how much my mom and step-dad struggled, even though they worked so hard. That understanding came later. But it also came with a feeling that I had seemingly insurmountable challenges ahead of me that I did not feel confident enough to overcome.

Like most people, my mom had strong beliefs that were shaped by the major events in her life. She believed that for a girl, a college education was the only way to protect herself from having a difficult life in case she ended up with a bad husband.

Having been married in Ecuador at the age of fifteen, my mom never finished high school. I was born three months before her eighteenth birthday and by the time she was twenty, she and my father were divorced. This led to some difficult times for my mother, including financially difficult times, which, of course, I don't remember but which she always recalled during my childhood. My mom (or so she tells me) needed to move somewhere where she could get a job despite having no education. Thus, my mother bravely moved to the United States with my sister and me in tow. I was only three. My sister, ten months younger.

The United States, of course, represented a better life, and my mom reminded me of that all the time. She used to tell me, "You need to go to college so in case you marry a bad man, you have a backup plan. You'll have something to fall back on so you don't have to put up with him. You see, then it's easier to get a good job." The gravity and sadness of her well-intentioned advice completely escaped the happy ten-year-old me, but I heard this message often enough growing up that by the time I was finishing high school, I knew college was the only way to go.

My mom remarried by the time I was six years old and shortly thereafter had my two younger brothers. That's how we had a family of six: my mom, my step-dad, me, my sister, and my two little brothers. This is the family I grew up with in Brooklyn, New York. My parents had many jobs, but mostly, my mom worked as a seamstress in several of the textile factories that existed in our neighborhood in the 1980s. My step-dad was a taxi driver for many years. Because my mom was a seamstress, she made many of our clothes as we were growing up, especially summer clothes, which were easier to make. The summer before I started high school, however, was the last time I would want to wear my mom's fashion creations.

That summer, I told my parents that I wasn't going to go to our local high school but instead was going to be attending Clara Barton High School near Prospect Heights. They asked me why, and I told them because I was going to be a doctor and Clara Barton was a high school for health professions. I had applied to go to this public school outside of my neighborhood all on my own, without asking them for permission. They asked how this happened and how was I going to get to a school that was far away. I told them that the New York City Transit Authority had bus and train passes for students, and I knew how to get them. I had it all figured out.

I don't think I really wanted to be a physician. It's just that, by the time I was in the eighth grade, I was already itching to get out of where I lived, though I certainly would not have been able to articulate why at that point. This was one way I could do it. Being a physician was an admired and respectable profession, so why not? After all, my grandmother had been a nurse in Ecuador. Without having anyone to provide me mentorship in this area of my life, being a physician

This place is wonderful and has the most hardworking and friendliest staff. Dr. Castilla is amazing, very knowledgeable and easy to talk to. They also have a very affordable payment plan that will work around your budget. I am so glad I found this place and can't imagine getting braces anywhere else. I'm incredibly thankful to Dr. Castilla and her team for giving me the smile I've always wanted.

—*Melanie C.*

seemed like a good ticket out. In my mind, it didn't matter that I knew nothing about being a physician and what it took to be one. My parents didn't really know anything about career planning and choosing schools. (Frankly, I didn't either.) So they went with it and were happy one of their kids wanted to go to college.

Going to Clara Barton High School was a defining event in my life. I was now going to school with kids whose parents owned homes or lived in nice apartments with soft carpet. (Yes, I thought carpet was the epitome of luxury.) No one in my neighborhood had anything but linoleum floors that covered the rotting wood underneath the hundred-year-old apartment buildings we were living in. Furthermore, many of my friends had their own bedroom. What? How rich *were* these people? Truthfully, they were all middle-class kids, not rich at all, but I was sharing my linoleum floor bedroom with all three of my siblings, so having my own bedroom seemed like a major luxury. This is what I wanted—my own bedroom and carpet and the job that would get it for me.

Once I started high school, I discovered that most of my classmates there wanted to go into nursing rather than medicine. This was often because it took so long to become a physician. I felt that way, too, once I learned what it took. When you're fifteen years old, finishing school at age thirty seems like a life sentence. There was also the fact that my adolescent self lacked any patience and appreciation for the journey. At that point, I wanted what I thought was success, sooner rather than later. I thought to myself, "I can't be broke till I'm thirty. My life will be almost over by then!" (Funny how thirty sounds young to me now.)

Going to Clara Barton High School was a defining event in my life.

You may be thinking I must have been the nerdiest and most overly serious kid in the tri-state area, but I really was like everyone else. I loved Paula Abdul and Bell Biv DeVoe, and like many girls in my school, I was obsessed with *Pretty Woman*. But then again, sometimes I wasn't like everyone else. I was constantly obsessed with my future and how I was going to make it better. I just had no clue how I was going to do it.

Soon after that, I discovered that I didn't have to make a decision. Around the time I was a junior, my parents decided to move to Columbus, Ohio, because it was *mas tranquilo* (Spanish for more peaceful) than Brooklyn, and the rent was so cheap we could move to a three-bedroom apartment. I would only have to share a room with my sister. But even the allure of getting closer to my own bedroom was not enough for me to want to leave New York. Not only did I have a limited black-and-white vision of success, I also had a limited black-and-white sense of identity. And that identity was of me as a New Yorker.

"But I'm from New York!" I protested with all the inflexibility of a sixteen-year-old.

"You're under eighteen, so you're coming with us," was the rebuttal.

I reluctantly moved to what I then referred to as "Cow-lumbus" (great city by the way). It was in Columbus, Ohio, where I eventually graduated from high school.

By the time I was a senior in high school, I was long done with the idea of being a doctor, but in my mind, that left me back at square one. What was I going to do? I was getting closer and closer to eighteen years of age and therefore time for me to go to college. One day, I went to the library (there was no Wikipedia then) and went to the career section. There, I gravitated toward books about engineering. I only saw my biological father once after moving to the United States, but I always heard so many stories about him (good and bad). He was a civil engineer and an architect, my mother had told me many times. I thought, maybe that's what I should do. After all, I could be an engineer after just four years in college. This was my new game plan.

One day, I was on the school bus going home after school when I sat next to a boy. He asked me if I had a boyfriend. That was not a conversation I wanted to have with him so I switched the subject and asked him if he had taken the ACT yet.

He said, "Nah man. That's just another standardized test. What, you wanna get into college or something?"

I said yes.

He replied, "Whatcha gonna do there?"

I told him I was going to major in engineering.

He said, "Do you even know what that is?"

Deeply offended, I replied, yes, I did. I had not only read up on it but my father was an engineer.

That conversation on that bus stuck with me forever. One, because I realized he was right. I didn't have the slightest idea what I was talking about. And two, because it fueled my drive like never before. Who was he to question my desire to go to college, even if I had no clue what I was going to be doing there?

My plan had always been to go to college, but it was for reasons different than fulfilling a career dream or studying a beloved subject. I wanted security. I wanted a good job. I wanted a better life. My senior year was a stressful time in my young life. I was in a new city and state, I didn't know what I wanted to do in college, and I also didn't know how I was going to pay for it. (Years later, my jaw would drop when some of my college classmates would tell me their parents were paying for their entire college.) I became disinterested and sometimes skipped school. I even skipped my senior yearbook picture day. I hated being in pictures and I hated my smile and I didn't want to be part of this stupid high school anyway. I entered a period in my adolescence where I became rebellious and argued with my mother. I decided I was going to go back to New York. So, taking my savings from my job at JC Penney, I bought a one-way Greyhound ticket to New York. I ran away. Just like that. But having nowhere to go, I ran to my grandmother's apartment. Hilarious looking back at it now. Who runs away to their grandmother's house?

My mom immediately went to New York. She never scolded me or told me to go back. She didn't have to. I knew she didn't suddenly go to New York because she was bored. It was understood. So back I went. Years later, I would recall that event as one her greatest displays of love for me.

After that, I decided that going to college in New York would be a great way to return to the life I had known before. Life had other plans for me, though. My guidance counselor had recommended that I apply to The Ohio State University, which is in Columbus. I flatly declined, but she wisely insisted. She said there was a full-tuition scholarship they had available and she felt pretty confident I had a chance of getting it. I had excellent grades in high school, so I can see why she thought this. What I didn't have then was a lot of self-confidence. Surely, I would never get this scholarship. But I applied to Ohio State and for the scholarship she recommended; if nothing else, to be polite. But one day I got two letters in the mail. One stated I had been accepted to The Ohio State University. The other letter stated I was in the final round of candidates for the full-tuition scholarship.

The day I went for the scholarship interview, I had to walk there because I had spent all my money on the outfit I was going to wear and because my mother had forgotten she was supposed to give me a ride and had gone off somewhere else with her friend. She didn't mean any harm, but I'll never forget that day. Even today, I remember what I wore to the interview. Not only because it was a hideous outfit, but also because I vividly remember sweating under my white blouse and my white pantyhose the entire time I walked to the interview. I walked for more than two hours, and I remember the relieving sensation of the cool air-conditioning I felt the moment I walked into the building.

Soon after the interview, I got another letter from Ohio State. The scholarship was mine. They had chosen me. I cried tears of joy. New York would not see me for at least a couple of years to come. I was now a Buckeye.

I quickly learned to love Ohio State, but there was definitely some culture shock I experienced when I got there. Someone had impelled me to apply to Ohio State, whereas many of my classmates were third-generation Buckeyes. I

Even today, I remember what I wore to the interview. Not only because it was a hideous outfit, but also because I vividly remember sweating under my white blouse and my white pantyhose the entire time I walked to the interview.

also still didn't know what my major would be. My advisors offered engineering as a good career for me. I was good at math and science, they said. I liked that I could get a job after only four years.

After taking a class for undecided students, I settled on welding engineering. Did I know anything about welding? Nope. But I was told that chemical engineering and welding engineering always ranked at the top of best-paying jobs with a bachelor's degree. So I chose welding engineering. Chemical engineering seemed too difficult. I wasn't sure I could do it. And that was that. My love for the subject was not considered. What I was going to actually enjoy doing in my life was not considered. The only consideration was, "Can I get a good-paying job?"

When I was nineteen, I got accepted into a summer internship at a General Motors plant in Pontiac, Michigan. I rented a room from a lady who had a house in Sterling Heights and spent the summer learning from manufacturing engineers. It was a traditionally masculine world that I had never seen before. Mostly male workers, auto parts, factories, assembly lines, etc. After spending one entire day in a blue-print room by myself organizing Mylar drawings, I thought of that kid on my school bus that day. I second-guessed my decision to do engineering. I wasn't sure if this would make me happy, even if I was good at it. The problem was, I didn't know what else to do. Furthermore, I had a scholarship I was NOT going to waste under any circumstances. So I continued with my welding engineering degree, but because several of my friends were on their way to medical school, I revisited that idea. Maybe medicine was for me after all? I stayed an extra year in college taking pre-med classes, just in case. This was a point in my life where I was really lost. I dreamed of a certain life, but I didn't know how to get there and be happy. I think, mainly, because I didn't know myself.

After five years of college, I graduated. I was three months shy of my twenty-third birthday. I felt a little burnt out from school and I had several job offers. Medical school was still in the back of my mind, but being eager to have an income, I decided to accept a manufacturing engineer position at Delphi Automotive Systems in Columbus. At the time, Delphi was a division of General Motors, but soon after split off from GM. The plant is now closed.

Having a good job provided some relief in the sense that, for the first time, I could buy for myself many of the things I could never buy before. I got a nice apartment (with a carpeted bedroom). And I got braces. The moment I had some money from my new post-college job, I landed in an orthodontist's office to get braces.

To most people in my life, this move seemed to come out of left-field. No one had ever really heard me complain about my smile. Even my mom was surprised. "Why did you get those?" she asked. "I don't remember your teeth being that bad."

"How can you say that?" I replied. I had asked her for braces once before. Besides, did she never notice the uni-fang I had on the upper left-hand corner of my mouth? Truth be told, I wasn't surprised she was surprised. I wasn't surprised anyone was surprised. As I mentioned before, I had never spoken to anyone about it. I hated my teeth, but like any pain in my life, it was something I kept inside, to myself. Now, everyone knew and it honestly felt better that it was out in the open. At least I was doing something about it.

I loved my orthodontist. He was so personable and funny. He always asked me about my life and would somehow remember things I had told him eight weeks before. Sometimes he would flex his arm muscles just to be goofy. I thoroughly enjoyed the whole process— even the dental work I had to get prior to starting treatment. Everyone I encountered in the dental field was very caring, and I felt like I was doing something for myself that wasn't related to school or my career. I used to run to the bathroom every morning to see where my teeth were at that day. I was looking and feeling better every day. Not until

I saw my smile improving did I ever realize what a negative effect my old smile had had on my self-esteem.

While I was happy with my newly developing smile, I was not happy with my job. I worked in a factory that had a lot of red tape and gave me very little meaningful interaction with other people. I decided that maybe I needed a different job somewhere else. Consequently, while in the middle of my orthodontic treatment, I accepted a job at a Ford Motor Company plant in Avon Lake, Ohio, just west of Cleveland. At the time, they assembled E-class vans and Mercury Villager and Nissan Quest minivans. Being unhappy at my job, I saw this as an opportunity to make a fresh start. New company, new city. I never left my orthodontist, though. Every time I had an appointment, I drove the two and a half hours it took to get from my apartment in West Lake to his office.

Meanwhile, some of my friends were getting into medical school. This is only relevant because even after taking the job at Avon Lake, I realized it was not the company—it was the job. I didn't like being an engineer in a manufacturing plant. The old idea of going to medical school resurfaced. I even signed up for the MCAT. Then I remembered a conversation I had had with one of the physicians who owned the apartment building I used to live in when I was in college. She had warned me not to go into medicine unless it was my passion. It was a long road and a challenging job. That's when I realized that I was

> *Everyone I encountered in the dental field was very caring, and I felt like I was doing something for myself that wasn't related to school or my career.*

just trying to go to medical school to escape engineering. I did love engineering itself, but I wanted to work in a completely different environment.

I wanted to help people, not assembly lines. A close friend of mine said to me, "Well, you can't stop talking about your teeth, have you ever thought of being a dentist?" That piqued my interest. Back to the library I went. (There was still no Wikipedia back then.) I researched everything I could find about being a dentist. I even called a West Lake dentist to ask if I could shadow him. He generously said yes, and I always try to remember his generosity when young people call my office requesting to job shadow.

I was still in braces when I started to consider dentistry as my future career, so I asked my orthodontist about it. "I'm thinking of going to dental school," I said.

He was so kind and encouraging and said: "I love my job. And I think you would love being a dentist."

Eight months later, I was accepted to The Ohio State University College of Dentistry and I thought I had hit the big time. I was braces-free by this point. I had a beautiful smile and I was going to be a dentist. My new plan: finish dental school and get a good-paying job at a private practice. See a recurring theme here?

I met a lot of great people in dental school, some of whom I am still friends with today. Many had big aspirations. From day one, some of my classmates told me they were going to be an endodontist, or an oral surgeon, or an orthodontist, or a general dentist owning their own private practice. I had never met so many confident people in my life. I was just happy I got in.

Dental school was the toughest time of my life, but also the greatest (I even met my husband, Eddy during this time). After I graduated, I moved to Dallas, Texas, to do a General Practice

Residency (GPR) at the Dallas VA Medical Center. When I was interviewing for GPR programs though, I was often told that my dental board scores were good enough to allow me to specialize. I never thought that was possible for me. I was twenty-nine years old now and not devoid of confidence, but I still thought some things were too "big" for me.

I lived in Texas with Eddy for five years practicing general dentistry. I enjoyed dentistry very much and it was during this time that I gained a lot of confidence. You see, getting a beautiful smile gave me the confidence to go to dental school—but helping others with their smile gave me the confidence to do anything I wanted. I thoroughly enjoyed helping my patients and this taught me to not focus so much on myself and instead to find fulfillment in helping others. I always joke that dentistry taught me all the communication skills I never learned in engineering school. It's kind of true. I had to be a caregiver now and provide empathy and comfort whenever needed. My job now involved not only science and medicine, but also relationship building. I was quite content.

From the time I started practicing as a general dentist, I started working with various orthodontists, because many of my dental implant patients needed braces before they could get implants. I also treated a lot of children who needed orthodontic treatment. I would often go to these orthodontic offices to discuss cases and what I saw in their offices was the missing piece of the puzzle in my professional life. Their offices were bona fide smile havens. They were fun, played young music, and were full of patients who were there because they wanted to be there. I said to myself, "These guys are having way more fun than I am!"

These orthodontists were changing the lives of their patients by giving them a beautiful smile. I saw a teenage girl sharing her prom dress photos with her orthodontist. I saw a mom hugging her son's orthodontist after his braces came off. One orthodontist office I visited had a corkboard full of letters and thank-you notes from patients and parents describing how orthodontic treatment had changed their lives. This brought me full circle because it was my quest for a beautiful smile that had inspired me to leave engineering and become a dentist. Why hadn't I thought of being an orthodontist before? Plus, I was an engineer. What better job for me than to be able to build little machines (braces) in people's mouths? I loved it. When I was in dental school, I had still been so caught up in my childhood fears of financial insecurity that I completely overlooked the fact that orthodontics was perfect for me. It was right there, literally in my face, all along and I never saw it.

But could I go back to college for a second time? I was already thirty-four years old and making a good living as a dentist. Wasn't that what I always wanted? It was a very difficult decision to make, but at the age of thirty-four, I decided to go back to school and become an orthodontist. It was the only time in my life that I made a career decision that was not based on economics. I finally gave myself permission to choose something strictly for the love of it, and I was finally confident enough to realize I deserved to dream this big.

What better job for me than to be able to build little machines (braces) in people's mouths?

My husband is a dentist and he says he knew he wanted to be a dentist since he was eleven years old. I never dared to dream that big. I barely knew what an orthodontist was when I pursued orthodontic treatment. I went in for a beautiful smile and came out with a career—the career of my life. It's like I always tell people, "I didn't look for orthodontics, orthodontics found me."

Chapter 2

A BEAUTIFUL SMILE
IS EVERYTHING

"A smile is happiness you'll find right under your nose."
Tom Wilson

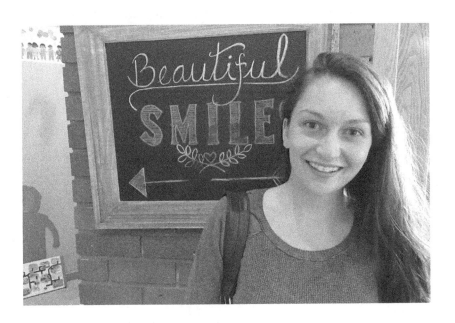

My friend Megan loves to giggle. She's kind of known for it. And it's not that she giggles for no good reason. She giggles when something is truly funny or when the irony of something brings her joy. But she does it for so long! She'll tell you something she thinks is funny all while simultaneously giggling. The result? Everyone around her starts to laugh or giggle as well, usually until she's done. It happens every time. Why? Because physiology is contagious.

If you're grumpy or rude, then you're likely to put others in a bad mood or even put them off. The same thing happens with laughter and smiling. What happens when you smile at someone? They smile back, of course. If for some odd reason you've never noticed this, you should try it today. Even babies know what to do. Smile at a baby and they will smile right back at you. (Unless they're hungry, of course, at which point no one can reasonably smile. I know I can't.)

Why does this happen? Because humans are social creatures.[1] Our brains have been shown to automatically and subconsciously mimic the facial expressions of others as a large component of emotional empathy. We do this regardless of what we verbalize. It's how we connect.[2] Body language has, after all, been shown to be the largest part of communication. Thank goodness. This is how I have successfully navigated my way around cities in Europe where I don't speak the language. Ordering food at a restaurant in Paris? Yes, it takes fifteen minutes, but I have a big smile on my face the whole time. I don't want to annoy anyone. The result? I get a smile in return (and a lot of patience and sympathy, too).

You may be thinking that you want a beautiful smile for yourself, not just to make babies smile. Well, you're in luck, because science

---

1   Jonah Lehrer, "The Mirror Neuron Revolution: Explaining What Makes Humans Social," *Scientific American*, https://www.scientificamerican.com/article/the-mirror-neuron-revolut.

2   Sarah Stevenson, "There's Magic in Your Smile: How Smiling Affects Your Brain," *Psychology Today*, June 25, 2012, www.psychologytoday.com/us/blog/cutting-edge-leadership/201206/there-s-magic-in-your-smile.

has shown that smiling increases your health and happiness, not just at the moment, but even in the long run.[3] So guess what? The more you smile, the healthier and happier you will be (that makes me want to smile). Research shows that a person's physiology or body language not only affects others around them, but it affects the individual as well. Try shaking your butt when you're grumpy and see how long you can stay grumpy. You can't do it! This is because emotions are created not only by our thoughts and our language, but also by our physiology. If you're depressed, you will have a particular body posture and body language that goes with it. Same thing when you're happy.

Science has shown that smiling increases your health and happiness, not just at the moment, but even in the long run.

How does the brain do this? When you smile, your brain releases signaling molecules called neuropeptides to the rest of your body.[4] These neuropeptides influence your brain, body, and behavior in many ways, including reducing stress, aiding sleep, and elevating your mood. There are other brain chemicals to enjoy as well. Give the world a big smile and your brain releases feel-good neurotransmitters, such as dopamine, endorphins, and serotonin. These chemicals calm your nervous system by lowering your heart rate and blood pressure. It's great to know that even when you skip out on going to the gym

---

3   Leo Widrich, "The Science of Smiling and Why It's So Powerful," *Buffer Blog*, April 9, 2013, https://blog.bufferapp.com/ the-science-of-smiling-a-guide-to-humans-most-powerful-gesture.

4   Eric Jaffe, "The Psychological Study of Smiling," *Association for Psychological Science*, December 2010, https://www.psychologicalscience.org/observer/ the-psychological-study-of-smiling/comment-page-1.

So glad this place was recommended to me a few years ago! It's been great. I love all the employees, they are super attentive to your needs, especially Dr. Castilla. Highly recommend to come here if you are in need of an orthodontist.

—*Joely H .*

(which I don't recommend doing), you can still work on your health by smiling away.

Need another reason to smile? How about being more attractive? That's enough reason for me, I'll tell you that. Turns out your smile is your best accessory. Studies have shown that people who smile are automatically viewed as more attractive, reliable, relaxed, and sincere. Seeing an attractive face can be considered a rewarding stimulus, and when a person sees a smiling face, the region of their brain that processes sensory rewards (called the orbitofrontal cortex) is activated significantly more than when viewing a non-smiling face.[5]

That is the magic and gift of a beautiful smile.

Smile Like a Boss: A Beautiful Smile Is the Key to Confidence

Now we know that smiling is good for your emotional well-being and is a major component of social interaction and our relationships with others. When you smile, you not only feel good, but you help others feel good. But how many of us will actually smile if we have gapped, bucked, or severely crooked teeth? Few things make me sadder than knowing someone is going through life without wanting to smile. I know what this feels like, because you will find very few pictures of me in high school or college with a smile on my face. Even in my college graduation picture, I didn't smile.

Today, being able to smile is even more important than ever. Children today are leading very public lives thanks to the Internet and social media. We are living in the era of selfies and YouTube videos. The pressure to look attractive or at least not be different,

---

5   J. O'Doherty et al., "Beauty in a Smile: The Role of Medial Orbitofrontal Cortex in Facial Attractiveness," *Neuropsychologia* 41 (2003), 147–155.

is greater than ever, as evidenced by the escalating levels of bullying now seen in schools. But it's beyond the schoolyard meanies. How will a child with crooked teeth be affected in college or after, when they have to go on job interviews? After all, a nice, relaxed smile during a job interview helps put others at ease and conveys a sense of calm, control, and most importantly, confidence. Today, job searching websites are littered with articles that describe the importance of smiling during a job interview. Smiling instills trust and convinces others that you are approachable and open—a team player, if you will.

How about dating? Confidence is sexy, and it is impossible to look, feel, and be confident if you hide your smile. Ever been on a date with someone who doesn't smile at anything you say or only smiles with their lips closed? Not only does it make you feel uncomfortable, it is almost impossible to connect. They may even come across as disingenuous. But someone who smiles big throughout a date? That person will come across as confident (and sexy). Smiling and confidence are a two-way street.

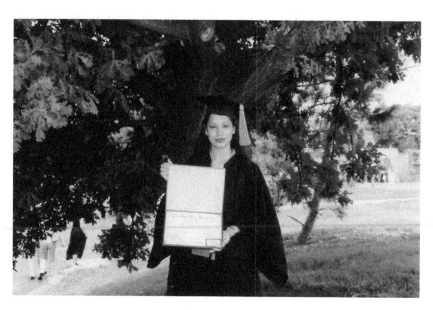

A Beautiful Smile Is a Healthy Smile

I think most people understand the immense social benefits of having a beautiful smile, but what I think a lot of people don't realize is that a beautiful smile is simply the result of a healthy smile and bite. When your teeth are healthy and fit well, they are beautiful. It's as simple as that. And aside from life happiness, amazing social skills, rock-star job interviewing, and confident dating, having straight, well-fitting teeth can also:

- **Help prevent gum disease.** Straight teeth are far easier to clean, which can help prevent gum disease, which is an inflammatory disease that has very serious health implications including increased risk of heart disease and diabetes.

- **Improved eating and nutritional health.** Teeth that fit well function better. Having teeth that don't meet or collide due to crowding results in poor chewing that can lead to digestion and nutrition problems.

- **Help you keep them longer.** Aligned teeth that fit well are more likely to last a lifetime. Not only are crooked, crowded teeth harder to clean (which can lead to cavities and gum disease), they also wear rapidly and prematurely, due to the fact that they collide during function. In cases of severe crowding, crooked teeth can also result in gum recession and increased sensitivity due to dental root exposure.

- **Decrease the risk of tooth injury from accidents.** Not only are crooked teeth harder to fit into a mouth guard, but protruding teeth are also more likely to chip or break. They simply stick out more.

- **Decrease the risk of jaw joint (TMJ) pain and headaches.** Crowded, ill-fitting teeth affect where and how you position your jaws, often resulting in chronic pressure that leads to headaches.

- **Improve your speech.** Crooked, protruding teeth are often the hidden cause of impaired speech that often affects school or job performance and self-esteem.

Some people put off orthodontic treatment—and they do so for many reasons: fear of pain, finances, and lack of understanding about the consequences. But as you can see, having a beautiful, healthy smile and bite is a huge component of a person's emotional, psychological, and physical well-being. The problems created by misaligned teeth and a poor bite don't just go away. They only get worse and harder to resolve as time goes on. I know I wish I had gotten my braces sooner.

Whatever is getting in your way of going after the smile of your life, I want to help you see that a beautiful smile is attainable. That is why I wrote this book—because a beautiful smile is everything.

Chapter 3

YOU'VE DECIDED.
NOW WHAT?

"May your choices reflect your hopes. Not your fears."
Nelson Mandela

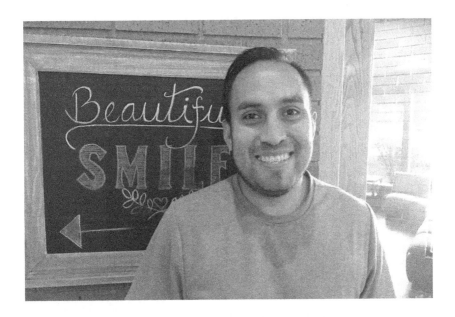

Desiree and her dad came in to our office after going to multiple consults. "Everyone has said surgery," Dad told us, "but surgery is not an option for us."

"I can definitely see how other doctors have said that, and indeed, that may be the best option for obtaining the most ideal results." I replied. I then proceeded to examine Desiree's bite and noticed that when her jaws came together in a natural position, she didn't have the large underbite she had as when she positioned her lower jaw to be able to chew. Desiree had two bites: her natural bite (which had no underbite) and her adapted bite, which caused her to go into an underbite so that she could chew.

I looked up at Dad. "Desiree's jaws are not as far off as they seem," I said. "I think I can do this without surgery."

Dad looked at me suspiciously at first but when I showed him Desiree's two bites, he understood. He understood very well. "No other orthodontist we saw realized she had two bites," he said. "I'm so glad we came here."

Listening is indeed an art, and it's one that every doctor should master. When deciding which orthodontist is right for you, you want to make sure you are selecting someone who is not only skilled, but someone who is also truly listening to your concerns and desires about your smile and experience. After all, everyone is unique. The concerns or desires you may have about your smile and treatment may not be the same as the other person in the reception area.

When Desiree and her dad came to my office, I could hear it in her dad's voice that he was serious. I understood. Surgery was not an option for them, and believe me, they had their personal reasons for this. They were not asking me to perform a miracle, but they were asking me to look for another solution. This prompted me not only to think critically when evaluating her case, but also to think outside the box. What could I do to make her smile better? Was there something I could be overlooking? Was there anything I could do to make her smile better or even correct it altogether? This was a difficult case, and if I was going to help her, then I needed to find a way to do it without surgery. Nearly three years later, Desiree has a beautiful smile and has become one of my favorite patients.

The decision to invest in orthodontic treatment for yourself or your child is a big one but following the excitement of that decision comes the sometimes-daunting decision of choosing the right orthodontist. You've decided, but now what? The Internet can be a great source, and we are lucky to be living in a time when we can review mounds of information and make a choice. Before the Internet, you just went to whoever your dentist referred you to or picked whoever had the nicest ad in the yellow pages. The flip side of this is that the gigabytes of information on the Internet can be overwhelming. My goal for this chapter is to provide you with a guide on how to choose not the best orthodontist (that is subjective), but the best orthodontist for you.

First, Is the Doctor a Specialist?

When my husband, Eddy, was a resident at the University of Tennessee Medical Center in Knoxville, he let his sister borrow his Acura when she went to visit him. Seems harmless enough, but in a twist of fate that only my sister-in-law could pull off, she ran over a blown tire on the road that caused his car's gas tank to tear. (I didn't even know a gas tank could tear.) Soon after getting over this major annoyance (he still remembers), Eddy went on a wide search for a mechanic. But, he was an underpaid hospital resident, so he chose the least expensive mechanic he could find. The problem? This mechanic usually worked on American cars. But money was an issue and Eddy needed his car back in working order urgently. The gas tank was repaired. All was good. Or so he thought. A few days later,

This is the place to go for friendly, professional, fun and affordable orthodontics. Dr. Castilla and her team are knowledgeable, approachable, and dedicated to fantastic care.

—*Katie P.*

when Eddy walked to his car in the parking lot, he noticed his car was leaking gas. Later, he discovered that the mechanic, not having much experience outside of American cars, had put a Honda gas tank into Eddy's Acura.

Now I realize that people are not cars and doctors are not mechanics, but I hope I'm making my point. You wouldn't trust your knee repair surgery to a family practitioner, or your diabetes treatment to a dermatologist. You would choose a specialist, and the right specialist at that. Your smile is no different. While there are amazing general dentists out there who can take great care of the health of your teeth and gums, your smile and bite is best cared for by an orthodontist. And an orthodontist is a specialist.

Up until they graduate from dental school, orthodontists and general dentists follow a similar educational path. But graduation is where orthodontists and general dentists go their separate ways. After graduation, dentists go on into private practice and begin treating patients, helping them take care of their teeth by performing fillings, crowns, veneers, etc. Orthodontics, however, is one of the nine dental specialties recognized by the American Dental Association. And because it is a specialty, orthodontists must complete two to three more years of full-time schooling. This additional training is called a *residency*, and it is during this training that orthodontists learn how to move teeth properly and correct bites using braces and/or clear aligners.

Additionally, orthodontists are also dentofacial orthopedists. Many people don't realize this, but the specialty is actually called Orthodontics and Dentofacial Orthopedics. As a dentofacial orthopedist, orthodontists also specialize in the guidance and normalization of facial growth and development, which occurs primarily during childhood. Being skilled in both areas, orthodontists are able to diagnose any misalignments in the teeth and jaws, as well as the facial structures, and can devise a treatment plan that integrates both orthodontic and dentofacial orthopedic treatments, if appropriate.

Bottom line, orthodontists specialize in creating beautiful smiles and are the most qualified doctors to do this. Orthodontists are the experts at choosing the best treatment options for you. It's what we do all day long. Day in and day out. When searching for a braces or clear aligner provider, the first thing you want to determine is whether the doctor is a specialist (an orthodontist) or not. One way you can determine this is to search for the American Association of Orthodontics (AAO) logo on their website. Only orthodontists can be members of the AAO. Or if you don't see it, call their office and ask if the doctor is an orthodontist and not a general dentist that also does some orthodontic treatment. Take it from me, I was a general dentist for five years and I can assure you that during that time (before I received my orthodontics training), I understood very little about orthodontics and how to properly move teeth.

Additionally, orthodontists are also dentofacial orthopedists. Many people don't realize this, but the specialty is actually called Orthodontics and Dentofacial Orthopedics.

> If you are considering orthodontic treatment by a general dentist, here are some questions that you may want to ask them:
>
> - Did you take a weekend course in orthodontics, or have you taken more extensive training?
> - How many cases like mine have you treated?
> - Did you treat your own children or did you refer them to an orthodontist?

General dentists are great at what they do, but very few are good at orthodontics. It's not because they're not good doctors. Most of them are great doctors. It's just that the vast majority don't have the training necessary in orthodontics to handle anything but the simplest of cases.

Do They Treat Adults?

Braces are not just for kids, and it's never too late for a healthy, beautiful smile. In fact, a recent study conducted by the American Association of Orthodontics (AAO) showed that adults are seeking orthodontic treatment in record numbers.[6] From 2012 to 2014, adults seeking treatment from orthodontists in the United States and Canada increased 16 percent, resulting in a record high of 1.4 million patients ages eighteen and older. The AAO estimates that 27 percent of orthodontic patients in the United States and Canada are adults.

---

6   "Smiles Are in Style: New Study Says Adults Are Seeking Orthodontic Treatment in Record Numbers," American Association of Orthodontics, AAO Press Releases, October 2013, http://couserorthodontics.com/smiles-are-in-style-new-study-says-adults-are-seeking-orthodontic-treatment-in-record-numbers.

But not all orthodontic offices treat many adults. Many focus primarily on children, especially orthodontic offices that are associated with a pediatric dental office. At Castilla Orthodontics, we are proud that 37 percent of our patients are adults. Our oldest patient is seventy-eight and she's fabulous. I particularly embrace adult treatment because I received my orthodontic treatment as an adult and have an affinity for older patients.

Adult orthodontic treatment is different from traditional, child orthodontic treatment. That is to say, adult patients have different and unique needs that children do not have. I will talk more about this in Chapter 6 but suffice it to say that if you are an adult looking to get a beautiful smile, make sure that your orthodontist of choice treats plenty of adults in their practice.

Just as technology has advanced our lives in so many other ways, so technology has also improved the design, shape, and function of today's modern braces.

Does the Office Offer the Latest Technology?

Just as technology has advanced our lives in so many other ways, so has technology also improved the design, shape, and function of today's modern braces. New technology produces better results, with fewer visits and shortened treatment times. Therefore, it is important that the office you choose offers the latest technology.

If the office is still using film x-rays, doesn't offer esthetic braces, or is still taking gooey impressions for Invisalign or other clear aligner systems, you may want to consider another office. At our office, we offer digital x-rays, clear braces, TADs (more on that in Chapter 4), laser treatments, teeth whitening, and the iTero digital scanner to eliminate gooey impressions for our Invisalign patients. We are constantly exploring the latest technology that can improve the comfort of our patients and speed up their treatment.

What Does Their Quoted Fee Include?

I understand that the fee is an important part of your decision. I didn't get orthodontic treatment until I was old enough to pay for it myself for this very reason. However, like everything else in life, you do get what you pay for.

A lot of offices offer what seem to be lower fees at first, but these fees are not all-inclusive. When comparing offices, be sure to ask about possible extra fees, such as for records, broken brackets, emergency visits, retainers, canceled appointments, Invisalign refinements (I'll explain what refinements are in Chapter 8), extra visits, or treatment that extends past the estimated treatment time. All these fees can add up—and then you would be paying the same or more than an office that had an all-inclusive fee and has better customer service. Additionally, if you are an adult patient, your orthodontist may require auxiliary appliances, such as Temporary Anchorage Devices (TADs), or tooth movement accelerators, such as Accele-Dent (more about this in Chapter 6). If this is the case, then make sure you ask if there will be an additional fee for these auxiliaries.

If you don't, you might have an experience like one of my patients. When Laura came to me, she had been at a corporate orthodontic office for five years and still had lots of spaces between her teeth. Needless to say, she was unhappy about this, but what finally "broke the camel's back" and caused her to leave that office and transfer to ours is all the extra fees she continued to pay. Five years in, she had already paid her treatment fee in full. However, the office required her to pay a $35 co-pay each time she went in for a braces adjustment appointment. One time, she left the office and soon after realized that one of her wires had been left a little long and was poking her. She couldn't go back that day due to her work schedule but called the office to schedule an emergency appointment so her pokey wire could be clipped. When she went back? Yep. They charged her another $35 co-pay. Fortunately, Laura is now in our office. Her case is now going well and her spaces are almost closed. With no co-pays.

Please be sure to read all the fine print when signing up for orthodontic treatment, and make sure you are clear about what you are getting for the fee you are paying. Pay attention to hidden fees and ask if there are any other possible charges that could come up later in treatment.

How Accessible Is the Office and How Easy Is it to Communicate with Them?

Ever called a professional office during business hours and they don't answer the phone, and it's not lunch time? Annoying, isn't it?

Everyone is busier than ever. You may be a busy professional or a busy parent—or, most likely, both! You want to make sure that when you try to reach your orthodontist's office, it doesn't take an act of congress. Pay attention to how they answer the phone when you call to schedule a consultation. Are they attentive? Do they put you on hold for a long time or, worse, more than once? If you call after hours or during lunch, do they call you back promptly? If there were issues in communicating with the office at the start, then there's a good chance that this will happen again.

At our office, it is almost impossible not to reach us. We have phones (with someone answering during lunch), but we can also be reached via email, text, and Facebook Messenger. I've responded to weekend texts myself to address emergencies such as pokey wires or loose brackets. If you can't reach us, then you may be dialing the wrong number.

Another thing to consider is the number of office locations. Having multiple locations can mean increased flexibility if you constantly travel all over your city or area, because then you can go to the location nearest where you happen to be. On the flip side, if the office has multiple locations but only one doctor, that means they are only at each location one or two days a week, tops, because they have to be at their other locations too. If you know you will only be able to go to one of their locations, ask about the doctor's and the team's availability. You may not want to be committed to an office location that only opens a few times a month.

Remember that you will be at this office for anywhere between twelve and twenty-four months. Make sure they are attentive to your needs and are easily accessible.

What Is the Culture and Reputation of the Office?

One of the keys to successful orthodontic treatment is developing a trusting relationship with the orthodontist and the office staff. That begins by understanding what the practice is about. The culture of the office is everything. Remember that you are about to enter a twelve- to twenty-four-month journey with these people. You want to make sure you feel comfortable, safe, and well cared for.

Additionally, it should be fun. I repeat: Orthodontics should be fun. When I was in braces, my orthodontist used to tell me jokes, ask me about my life and job, played fun music, and his team always had a smile on their face. These are memories I will cherish forever.

Fortunately, it is very easy to figure out what the culture of the office is like. When you first call to schedule an initial consultation,

Orthodontics should be fun.

are they excited to receive your call? Is the receptionist polite, professional, and friendly? Does she ask about your concerns? When you get to the office, pay attention to the team. Are they dressed professionally? Do they greet you right away or do they not even notice that you walked in the door and have been waiting in the reception area for ten minutes? Does the clinical assistant that takes your photos and x-rays talk to you in a friendly, professional manner? Does she explain everything she is about to do so you feel comfortable and informed?

How about the office itself: Is it clean? Do they offer free Wi-Fi? Do they play fun music? Does the team seem happy and do they seem to be enjoying themselves? Do they offer fun contests and events for your child? Do they have a rewards program for kids? Is this a place you can see yourself coming to for the next couple of years?

Another way to get a feel for the office culture as well as their level of customer service is to research their reputation. Read the comments of their Google, Facebook, and Yelp reviews. What do the patients praise the most? Any major complaints? There's usually a consistent theme in an office's reviews. You can also ask your dentist or hygienist if they have heard of the office you are considering visiting.

The dental world is a small world and many dental professionals in a town either know each other or at least know of each other. Finally, ask your friends and neighbors what they've heard.

At our office, our patients are treated like family. We love our patients! Our goal is to change our patients' lives by transforming their smiles and we are honored to be part of their journey. Orthodontic treatment is a journey and we want to be our patient's cheerleaders along the way, encouraging them however we can. This is evident in our online reviews, in the way our friendly team interacts with our patients, and in the many referrals we get from our wonderful patients.

What Happens After Orthodontic Treatment Is Complete?

Once you get that beautiful smile, you want to make sure that it stays that way. After all, regardless of where you choose to go, orthodontic treatment is a big investment of your time and finances. Like most offices, we advocate lifetime retainer wear at night. It's the only way teeth stay the way they were when your braces came off. However, life happens. Retainers get lost or are simply forgotten due to other things in your life. Sometimes, teeth shift a little even with retainer wear. This is rare but can happen, especially if there was a severely rotated tooth to begin with, and often requires a change in retainer type.

Regardless of the reason for relapse (shifting), you want to get all the details of what would happen if your teeth did shift and needed correction. If it's through no fault of your own, does the office guarantee their results? We do. What if it is your fault? Maybe you lost your retainers and couldn't get back in to the office because you were backpacking through Europe. Now your teeth have shifted a little. What happens now? Make sure you understand the costs associated with fixing minor relapse.

In our office, we offer two programs to ensure our patients smiles stay as beautiful as we left them when the braces came off. One is our Lifetime Retainer Program, which allows patients to get replacement retainers at a very low cost. The other is our Guarantee My Smile program, where, for a small monthly fee, we will put braces back on until you are happy with your alignment again. It doesn't matter what the reason was—you lost your retainer, you simply forgot to wear it, or you accidentally stepped on it. Either way, we will put your braces back on until you are happy, and then we take them off. No big contract or big down payment. Just a small monthly fee.

Do They Offer Flexible Financing?

There are many reasons why patients hold off on starting orthodontic treatment for themselves or for their child, and finances is one of the biggest. Yes, orthodontic treatment can be a big investment. And for good reason. Just think of all the visits you will make to your orthodontist during your treatment, and everything that it will take to get your smile looking first class. But a big investment does not have to equate to lack of affordability.

Regardless of the total treatment cost, there are ways to make orthodontic treatment affordable. Most offices offer some type of in-house financing, but not all of them offer options such as low or zero down payment or financing extended beyond treatment time. If flexible financing is an important consideration for you, make sure to ask about in-house financing options. There are also third-party companies out there, such as Care Credit, that can help you finance your treatment. However, be careful to read the fine print with these contracts. Often times, the interest rates are really high or the penalties for a late payment are very steep. My personal recommendation is to avoid these third-party finance companies if at all possible. There are plenty of orthodontic offices out there that offer flexible in-house financing with zero or very minimal interest. I know we are one of them!

A final note of caution: Beware of offices that offer deeply discounted prices. These offices still have to be able to make a profit, so to give you those low prices, they often have to use cheap materials and cut corners wherever possible—including with customer service. You get what you pay for. Remember that this

> *Beware of offices that offer deeply discounted prices.*

is an investment in the smile of your life. Put your smile in good hands and be confident that with a little research, you can find a quality office that will make the investment affordable for you.

Selecting an orthodontist is a personal choice. Their office culture, availability, customer service, location, and financing options all play a role. A great orthodontist for you may not be a great orthodontist for me. And that's okay. The main thing is that you know what to look for.

Next, you get to decide on what treatment option is best for you. And just like selecting an office, this is also a personal choice.

Chapter 4

MY BRACES ARE NOT YOUR BRACES

"It's not hard to make decisions once you know what your values are."
Roy E. Disney

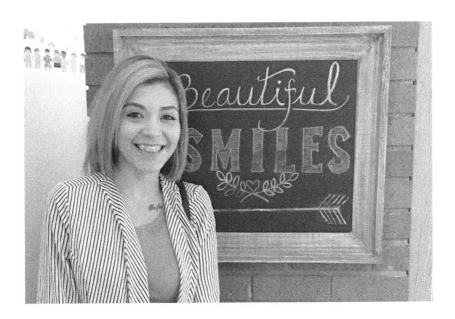

A couple of years ago, my husband and I went to the Dominican Republic for a family trip with my cousin, my brothers, and their respective families. The oldest of my two brothers had chosen the resort where he and the rest of the clan would stay. Due to my busy schedule and desire to be near my family, I decided to book a room in the same resort that they were staying in. My thoughts were along the lines of: "Sweet! I don't even have to plan this." So I handed over my credit card and our rooms were promptly booked at the same resort.

Punta Cana, Dominican Republic, is a beautiful town and the resort we stayed at was fantastic. The best part? Vacationing with my family, something I rarely get to do. But was this beautiful resort the choice my husband and I would've made if we were traveling alone? Not really. The resort we were at was very large—a veritable campus. We prefer smaller, more intimate resorts. We also like adult-only resorts, as we don't have children of our own. While having lots of activities within the resort was important to my brothers, Eddy and I like to venture outside of resorts and get a taste of local life. I could go on and on, but I think I'm making my point here—different strokes for different folks. Was there anything wrong with the resort we went to? Absolutely not. It was a great place and the people working there were so nice. It just was not what we would've elected on our own.

> *When it comes to your orthodontic treatment, it's important that you choose the braces that are right for you and for no one else.*

Braces are no different. (Seriously, only I could compare braces with resorts in the Dominican Republic.) When it comes to your orthodontic treatment, it's important that you choose the braces that are right for you and for no one else. You are an individual, with a unique personality, lifestyle, and taste. And today, you have more options than ever before. My goal is to provide you with an overall picture of the choices you have, to give you a springboard for doing your research and asking questions when you go to your orthodontic consultation.

What are the main types of braces?

While there are many treatment options available, it is important to understand that there are basically just two main types of braces available:

- fixed braces that are glued to your teeth and cannot be removed, and

- removable braces (clear aligners).

Everything else is a variation of these two main categories.

How Braces Work

Braces, including removable braces, work by applying light, continuous pressure over a period of time to slowly move teeth in a specific direction and toward an improved position within the jaw bone.

With fixed braces, the source of this light pressure is actually the wire that goes inside each bracket. Fixed braces can be made out of metal, or from tooth-colored ceramic for a less-visible look. Basically, the braces, also known as brackets, are bonded (glued) to each tooth. Each bracket has a little slot where the wire is inserted and then tied to each bracket so the wire doesn't fall out. With traditional, fixed braces, these ties (also called o-rings, o-ties, or elastic ligatures) can be silver or clear to match your braces, or you can select from a myriad of fun colors. The o-ties are changed at every adjustment appointment,

The staff is the nicest staff I've ever had. They are funny, sweet, and friendly. They are very organized, and you can earn or win stuff. I love this orthodontist and I would never go to a different one.

—*Torie P.*

so you can try a different color each time. Not all fixed braces need o-ties, though. Some fixed braces have been designed with built-in doors that close over the wire, "trapping" it inside their slot. Because of these built-in little doors, these braces don't need o-ties to tie the wire in and are, therefore, called self-ligating braces. Whether your braces need o-ties or are self-ligating, if your teeth are crooked or out of alignment, the wire must be displaced and gently pushed into each bracket because, while your teeth may be crooked, the wire is not. Because the wire wants to recoil back to its original shape, it brings the teeth with it. It's actually a little more complex than that, but that is the simple explanation of how fixed braces work.

With removable braces or clear aligners (e.g., Invisalign), it is not much different. A source of light, continuous pressure is still needed. The difference is that the pressure comes from wearing a series of aligners (sometimes called trays) that look like clear retainers but apply the light, continuous pressure needed to move your teeth. These clear aligners are changed out one or two times per week (usually one time per week) to a new, slightly different aligner. Basically, you wear an aligner that, over the course of one or two weeks, moves your teeth to a slightly different position. Once this small movement is complete, you switch to the next aligner the following week, and this new aligner will gently push your teeth into the next slightly different position. Thus, as you go through each aligner, your teeth gradually move into a more aligned and improved position.

One thing that is important to mention about clear aligners, especially Invisalign, is that unless your case is simple, you will almost certainly have at least a few attachments. What are these? Quite simply, attachments are tooth-colored ridges made of dental composite resin, a material very similar to what your dentist uses for tooth-colored fillings, that are bonded or glued to certain teeth, like braces. They come in different shapes and sizes and are only bonded on certain teeth—usually the ones that require a more difficult movement. The attachments are used as anchor points or "tooth grabbers" for teeth that need extra retention either because of their size and shape, or because of the difficulty of the movement needed. The attachments simply click into the aligners when you put them on.

What Is Important to You?

A lot of the information you will find in other books or on the Internet tries to help patients decide what kind of braces they should get by making a list of braces and then explaining the pros and cons of each braces type. I think this is a very appliance-centric approach with too much focus on the orthodontic appliance itself. Instead, I've decided that since you are reading this book to learn about the best options for yourself or your child, it is best to describe each type of braces within the context of what you, the patient, value. Thus, I have made a list of the most important aspects of orthodontic treatment that many of my patients ask me about when they come to my office for a consultation. And I've worn both traditional braces and Invisalign, so I can give you both the doctor and patient perspective.

Removability

As I mentioned, removability is the main difference between fixed braces and removable braces. Fixed braces are bonded to your teeth and stay on your teeth for the entire length of your treatment. In a sense, they are more of a "set it and forget it" type of braces. You cannot remove them to eat or to take a selfie. Thus, you will likely spend a little more time cleaning your teeth with fixed braces since you have to work around the brackets and the wires. On the plus side, braces only work when they are on your teeth, so if you think you or your child will forget to wear the "braces" (aligners), fixed braces may be best for you.

Clear aligners are removable braces and the most popular brand is Invisalign. There are other clear aligner systems out there, of course. These include systems like Clear Correct and MTM. But thanks to advances in their technology and some very clever marketing, Invisalign has become somewhat of a household name, especially in the dental world. Indeed, Invisalign is, by far, the leader in the clear aligner market.

If you actually wear them for the required twenty-two hours a day, you will find that there are some great advantages to being able to remove your braces. One

On the plus side, braces only work when they are on your teeth, so if you think you or your child will forget to wear the "braces" (aligners), fixed braces may be best for you.

of them is cleaning your teeth. Without brackets on every tooth and a wire connecting all of them, it is much faster and easier to keep your teeth clean. Anyone who has ever handled a floss threader can attest to this. That being said, I have patients in fixed braces with great oral hygiene and patients in Invisalign with whom we have to constantly review the importance of brushing and flossing. Some people keep their teeth clean and some people just don't. However, when you wear Invisalign, you will very likely have attachments and you do have to spend a little extra time cleaning around them, so it's not like Invisalign is a free ride, either. In the end, though, it is overall easier and quicker to clean your teeth with Invisalign or other clear aligner systems.

Another advantage of Invisalign and other clear aligners is that they can potentially reduce unplanned ("emergency") visits to the orthodontist. Since aligners can be removed for eating, you can pretty much eat anything you want, with no concern about breaking your braces. It is a lot harder to break off a properly bonded attachment than a bracket.

Bottom line: You need to take a good look in the mirror and have an honest conversation with yourself when deciding between removable and fixed braces. Without a doubt, Invisalign can provide excellent results with minimal, if any, sacrifices in your diet and with greater ease of cleaning your teeth. I've treated tons of Invisalign cases that have resulted in beautiful smiles. These patients were very disciplined and found wearing the aligners to be easy once they got used to them. However, if you are a heavy snacker, or sip on coffee for two hours each morning, Invisalign may not be right for you. Same goes if you have a job as a chef or a food critic, or if you have a teenager who can't keep track of his eyeglasses to save his life. Invisalign can give you a lot of flexibility, but with that, you or your child must have the discipline to wear the aligners the required number of hours or they will simply not work.

Visibility

I think it's important to address the difference between visibility and esthetics. "Visibility" is objective, while "esthetic" is subjective. After all, beauty is in the eye of the beholder, so I take issue with clear aligners or fixed ceramic braces being called "esthetic braces." Ask the twelve-year-old little girl I just put metal braces on, who is grinning from ear to ear about how cool her braces look and is on her cell phone telling her bestie about the awesome purple color she just chose for them. Believe me, those metal braces are esthetic to her! But for others, esthetic does in fact mean "less visible."

Fortunately, there are multiple options to choose from if you want your orthodontic treatment to be lower key. One option is a clear aligner system, such as Invisalign. Even with attachments on your front teeth, Invisalign is still less visible than ceramic braces and is virtually undetectable in photography. I recently wore Invisalign for about five months to correct some minor tooth relapse that occurred after I stopped wearing my retainer. (Please don't be like me.) As the owner of an orthodontic practice, I often get photographed for social media and advertisements and when I was in Invisalign treatment, you could hardly see my attachments or aligners on any of the photographs that were taken of me during that time. However,

Fortunately, there are multiple options to choose from if you want your orthodontic treatment to be lower key

as I stated before, you have to make sure that you wear your aligners as directed. If you don't think you will, then fixed, ceramic braces may be the better option for you, since they are still a lot less visible than metal braces, especially from a distance.

In the past, one of the objections to ceramic braces has been that the clear o-ties can stain in between adjustment appointments, thus decreasing the esthetics of the ceramic braces. This can especially happen if you eat or drink a lot of staining foods, such as coffee, wine, mustard, etc. Today, we have pearl-colored o-ties that don't stain nearly as much as the clear ones, but if you don't want to deal with staining o-ties at all, there are now ceramic self-ligating braces where the bracket "door" or "gate" is completely clear. As you may remember, self-ligating braces don't need o-ties at all.

If your desire is complete invisibility or you want less visibility than ceramic braces but you know you will be inconsistent at wearing aligners, then you may want to consider lingual braces. The term "lingual" comes from the Latin for tongue, "lingua," so—you guessed it—lingual braces are on the tongue side of your teeth. The best-known system is called Incognito, but there are others. Lingual braces have actually been around for a while and there have been a lot of technological improvements for this type of treatment, especially in terms of customization to the individual patient. Nevertheless, with the advent of clear aligner therapy, such as Invisalign, and material strength improvements for ceramic braces, the demand for lingual braces has decreased over the years. Today, it is more popular in Europe than it is in the United States. Lingual braces do bring the best of both worlds for those that want minimum or no visibility, but also don't have the discipline or personality to remember to wear aligners for twenty-two hours a day.

However, before considering lingual braces, there are several disadvantages you should know about. For one, this type of treatment can be technically challenging for any orthodontist, since people don't exactly have gobs of space on the tongue side of their teeth. Therefore, it may prove difficult to find an orthodontist who offers it, especially in smaller cities where the demand for this type of treatment is low. In large cities, such as Los Angeles and New York, lingual braces are far more common, especially among executive business people and celebrities. It has been said that Miley Cyrus wore lingual braces, and I know that the DJ (and awesome sidekick) on the *Ellen DeGeneres Show*, tWitch, also wore them. Finally, this type of treatment will be much more expensive than the traditional braces that are bonded to the front of your teeth, so if cost is an important consideration for you, this may not be the best option. There are a couple of other disadvantages that I will discuss in the next sections, but despite these, this is still the treatment of choice for those that want complete invisibility.

Comfort

Whether you choose traditional braces or Invisalign, there will be an adjustment period when you first start orthodontic treatment. Most people adjust within the first week or two. If you're wearing traditional braces, your lips and cheeks will need at least a week to adjust to rubbing up against the braces, especially when you are speaking. If you are considering lingual braces, please know that the adjustment period may be longer, because with this treatment all of your braces are facing your tongue and this can cause multiple sores on your tongue, especially in the beginning. Lingual braces can also give you a little bit of a slurred speech, especially if tongue sores develop.

With Invisalign or other clear aligners, your tongue will spend the entire first week rubbing up against the edges of the aligners until it learns to stop doing it. After the adjustment period, orthodontic treatment will pretty much feel normal. That being said, many patients, especially adults, do find Invisalign to be more comfortable than braces. Certainly, with Invisalign there is no risk of pokey wires or brackets coming loose. Also, with the aligners in, the attachments feel smooth compared to braces. If you feel your mouth is sensitive, clear aligner treatment may be the best option for you.

Lifestyle

People are getting busier than ever and I think lifestyle is an important consideration when choosing braces. If you are a super-busy professional who has a difficult time getting off of work, please consider Invisalign—unless you know you won't wear the aligners. Braces patients come in for check-ups at six- to ten-week intervals, while Invisalign patients come in at ten- to fifteen-week intervals. Additionally, the risk of unplanned visits for things such as pokey wires (though at our office we take great care to avoid those) or broken braces is almost nil. It's not just adults who are busy. In our office, we have some teens with sports and extracurricular activity schedules that rival the schedule of any busy adult. If your teen is so busy you feel like a "momager," Invisalign may be the option for them.

If you are a super-busy professional who has a difficult time getting off of work, please consider Invisalign—unless you know you won't wear the aligners.

If your teen participates in a high-contact sport, Invisalign can also make it easier for them to wear a mouth guard. And the fact that there are no braces to break off during a football game is also a plus.

On the flip side, traditional metal braces are a big source of individual expression for many patients, especially kids and teens who have a lot of fun picking different colors to match their mood, the holidays, or their school colors. Additionally, while I have had teens who do a great job wearing their Invisalign aligners, I've also had parents tell me that they know that their particular teen will not be responsible enough to remember to wear the aligners as they're supposed to. As one mom confided, "Doctor, I've already had to drive to her school twice this week to bring her her eyeglasses. And she needs those to see!"

Length of Treatment

The length of treatment is primarily determined by the details and complexity of the individual patient's case, as well as by the patient's compliance level. There are a lot of claims being made out there that Invisalign is faster or self-ligating braces are faster, but to that I say, what does it matter if someone is treated with Invisalign if the doctor is not very experienced with it? Will it be faster? The treatment will not be faster with Invisalign if the doctor does not have experience with it.

Also, some cases, due to their nature, may be faster with Invisalign, whereas others have the potential to be slower with Invisalign. Therefore, it would be incorrect to make a generalized statement that Invisalign is faster than fixed braces across the board. For example, Invisalign tends to be more successful at treating open bites, where the front teeth don't meet, than it is at treating deep bites, where the front teeth overlap excessively in the up-and-down direction. It doesn't mean a deep bite can't be treated with Invisalign. I've successfully treated many deep bites with Invisalign. However, it does mean that treatment of a deep bite has a better chance at going faster with fixed braces. The opposite is true with open bites. Invisalign will often treat open bite cases faster than will braces. Like I said, it all depends on the case.

Similar claims are sometimes made by some providers about fixed, self-ligating braces. These claims include decreased treatment time with self-ligating braces due to decreased friction between the wire and the brackets, as well as other reasons. However, the existing research in the orthodontic literature is inconclusive about this claim.[7] There are just too many factors involved in treatment time. I would personally beware of any provider that claims they need some special bracket to make their treatment go faster or better. There are technologies that can speed up orthodontic treatment, and I'll review those in Chapter 6, but barring the use of super-cheap, low-quality braces, the type of braces you choose will not necessarily speed up your treatment or make it any more efficient. I'm not saying that it's not important to pick the best type of braces for your or your child's particular case. But, there are multiple other factors that affect the length of treatment, including the type of bite, physiological factors (some people's teeth move faster than others), patient compliance, and the experience of the provider with your type of case and the type of braces selected.

Everyone is truly unique—not just with their teeth and bite, but also in their preferences, their lifestyle, and their personality. You know yourself better than anyone else, and your orthodontist will know your particular case as well. Together with your orthodontist, you can make an informed decision about which braces are best for you or your child. No one else.

7   Padhraig S. Fleming and Ama Johal, "Self-Ligating Brackets in Orthodon-
     tics," *Angle Orthodontist* 80, no. 3 (May 2010): 575–584, https://doi.
     org/10.2319/081009-454.1; Stephanie Shih-Hsuan Chen et al., "Systematic
     review of self-ligating brackets," *American Journal of Orthodontics and Den-
     tofacial Orthopedics* 137, no. 6 (June 2010): 726.e1–726.e18, https://doi.
     org/10.1016/j.ajodo.2009.11.009.

Chapter 5

SOMETIMES YOU HAVE TO JUMP IN EARLY

"Timing in life is everything."
Leonard Maltin

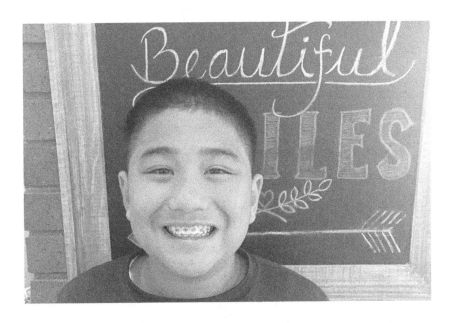

If controversy could ever be found in the field of orthodontics, it would be found in the topic of early orthodontic treatment (also known as interceptive treatment, or Phase 1

Treatment). This is because most people don't understand why a young child under ten years of age would ever need braces. The common belief is that a child needs to lose all their baby (primary) teeth before they are ready for orthodontic treatment. This leads to misunderstandings and misconceptions about why an orthodontist would put braces on a seven-year-old child. Is it because the child really needs it or is the orthodontist "greedy" and will put braces on anyone? Also, what happens when a young child is done with Phase 1 braces but still has baby teeth left?

Let me address the idea of the "greedy" orthodontist first. There are bad apples in *every* profession. This is true in any industry.

The American Association of Orthodontics (AAO) recommends that each child have their first orthodontic visit by the age of seven

Thankfully, most people are honest, and that includes orthodontists. Orthodontists have nothing to gain and everything to lose by getting a reputation for doing needless and unnecessary treatment. Our practices depend on referrals and the good will of our communities. In my practice, Phase I or early treatment patients make up 10 percent of my practice, and most children do receive comprehensive (single-phase) orthodontic treatment at a later age.

As far as what happens after early treatment, I will explain that later in this chapter. Let's just say that, often, if early treatment was done, a second treatment (called Phase 2) is usually needed later.

When is the best time to start orthodontic for your child? It depends. Sounds like a cop-out answer but, in fact, every child is unique, even when they are the same age and gender. This makes sense, right? Ever notice how some twelve-year-old girls look like they're nine and others look like they are juniors in high school? The teeth and jaws are no different in their variability.

The American Association of Orthodontics (AAO) recommends that each child have their first orthodontic visit by the age of seven, and I agree. This is because by age seven there has been sufficient jaw development and enough permanent teeth have erupted for an orthodontist to be able to identify whether there are any problems developing. This is important because some orthodontic problems are simply easier to correct at an earlier age. Thus, early screening can reduce the complexity of treatment later on. Furthermore, there are certain orthodontic problems that simply cannot be resolved past a certain age without the aid of surgical treatment.

What can you expect when you take your young child for an orthodontic evaluation? There are several main things an orthodontist will evaluate:

- Are the jaws developing normally?
- Is there sufficient room for the permanent teeth to grow in on their own?
- Are the teeth growing in correctly?
- Are there any crossbites?
- Are there any extra or missing teeth?

There are three possible outcomes from an orthodontic evaluation:

1.   Your child has an orthodontic problem that would benefit greatly from early intervention or treatment. If this is the case, the orthodontic treatment is split into two phases: Phase 1 and Phase 2. Phase 1 will address only the issue(s)

Dr. Castilla has been amazing to both my children and has continually worked to better their smiles. She is warm and compassionate toward their needs and listens to what the patient says. She also spends extra time whenever needed to make sure that her patients walk out happy and comfortable with their mouths. I would recommend her to anyone that is looking for orthodontic work.

—*Mark C.*

that is best treated at an early age, and the treatment can last between nine and eighteen months.

After Phase 1, your child will go into a "resting" period during which the orthodontist continues to see them at certain intervals to monitor their growth and development, as well as identify the best timing to start Phase 2. Phase 2 usually happens a year or even over two years after Phase 1 is completed. During Phase 2, the remaining orthodontic treatment is completed. Phase 2 treatment is usually of shorter duration and is less complex because the major issues were addressed in Phase 1.

2. Your child will benefit from orthodontic treatment but now is not the ideal time. In this scenario, the orthodontist has identified issues that will benefit from correction but recommends waiting. In this case, your child will typically be placed "on recall" (or in our office, our Pre-Orthodontic Guidance Program), where his or her growth and development will be monitored by the orthodontist every six months to make sure the orthodontic issues don't change for the worse, and to help the orthodontist identify the best time for your child to start their single-phase, comprehensive orthodontic treatment. Sometimes, even though Phase 1 treatment is not needed, removal of one or two baby teeth with your general or pediatric dentist is recommended at the time of the evaluation. Depending on the case, an appliance called a *space maintainer* may be needed to hold the space of the baby tooth that was removed.

3. It is not certain that your child will need any orthodontic treatment at all. In this case, your child will also be placed

in the office's recall program to monitor their growth and development and to make sure nothing changes. If it doesn't then your child is one of the very few kids with perfect teeth. Congratulations! If things do change, then at least it will be caught early and you will be well informed.

Types of Issues That Are Typically Addressed in Phase 1 (Early) Treatment

To help you understand why Phase 1 treatment may be needed, I have created a list of things that are commonly treated in Phase 1.

Through various treatments, including orthopedic jaw widening and/or strategic removal of certain baby teeth, severe crowding in a young child can be treated and potentially prevent impacted teeth.

Severe Crowding

When crowding is severe, the permanent teeth may not develop in their correct place and thus may have trouble growing in. Sometimes, crowding can be so severe that if left untreated, one or more teeth never make it in on their own. When this happens, the tooth is said to be *impacted*. This results in a more-complex and longer orthodontic treatment later on, because the child will then require an "exposure" surgery by an oral surgeon who surgically exposes the impacted tooth and bonds (glues) a small gold chain to it so that the orthodontist can slowly and over time "pull it" into the mouth in conjunction with braces and other orthodontic appliances. Through various treatments, including orthopedic jaw widening and/or strategic removal of certain baby teeth, severe crowding in a young child can be treated and potentially prevent impacted teeth.

Large Discrepancy or Difference between the Development of the Jaws

The growth and development of the jaws is a complex subject, but I will summarize it. For the teeth to fit together properly, the upper and lower jaws must be positioned in a certain relationship; both in a front-to-back direction and in a side-to-side direction. Additionally, each jaw must be of a certain size in relation to the other jaw. The human body allows for a certain range of variability in the relationship between the jaws; both in terms of position and size. However, there is a point where the difference in size and/or position is so big, that the teeth cannot fit together without orthodontic and dentofacial orthopedic treatment.

Orthopedic treatment, which involves guidance of the growth and development of the jaws, is primarily accomplished in the upper jaw because, unlike the lower jaw, which is one continuous bone, the upper jaw is composed of two halves that are, in children, connected to each other by soft tissue. That is, the two parts of the upper jaw (right and left) are not fused in children. It's kind of like a baby "soft spot" in the head of an infant. Infants have "soft spots" because the bones of their little skulls haven't fused yet. The bones of a young child's upper jaw haven't fused yet, either. This changes with time, and as the child gets older, the two halves of the upper jaw begin to fuse more. That is why growth guidance of the upper jaw is easier and more successful in young children under age ten. In fact, there are certain jaw size and position discrepancies that are severe enough that if they don't get treated properly at an early age, can lead to needing jaw surgery to reposition the jaws so that the teeth can properly fit.

Jaw size and position discrepancies can lead to skeletal crossbites and/or functional shifts. In a correct, healthy bite all of the lower teeth fit inside of the upper teeth. A *crossbite* is the term used when this relationship is reversed. That is, when the upper teeth fit inside of the lower teeth. Not all crossbites are the same and some are solely due to incorrectly positioned teeth, which is called a *dental crossbite.* Other crossbites are caused due to differences in the size and position of the jaws. These are called *skeletal crossbites. A functional shift* is when the child cannot get their teeth to fit together for chewing when they close down with their jaws in their natural position, so they shift their lower jaw in one or more directions so their teeth can come together and they can chew (function).

Dental Crossbites

As I mentioned, a dental crossbite is a crossbite that results from incorrectly positioned teeth or crowding and is not necessarily related to large differences in jaw size and position. Unlike skeletal crossbites, which involve an entire section of the jaw or even sometimes the entire jaw, dental crossbites are usually limited to one or two teeth. Many dental crossbites do not need to be treated right away but others, in particular those between the front teeth, can lead to gum recession of the lower front tooth that is in crossbite. This is because as the child bites down, the upper tooth, being inside or behind the lower one, "pushes" the lower tooth partly out of the lower jaw bone. This, in turn, can lead to gum recession. Gum recession, or the "peeling" away of the gum from the tooth, can be difficult to correct later on and often requires surgery by a periodontist. For this and other reasons, such as accelerated tooth wear, certain dental crossbites should be corrected as soon as they are identified.

Severe Protrusion

Protrusion (sometimes called "buck teeth") is the term used for upper teeth that protrude or extend too far forward in relation to the lower teeth. Protrusion is usually the result of a problem with the development of the upper and lower jaws, but it can also be the result of oral habits such as thumb sucking. A little protrusion can often wait to be treated at a later age, but severe protrusion, which can lead to difficulty in closing of the lips over the teeth, increased risk for tooth injury or trauma, chewing difficulties, and self-esteem issues from bullying at school, is best corrected early.

> *I have never had a parent who brought their child in for treatment of severe protrusion not tell me that their child was being bullied because of it.*

Bullying by other children breaks my heart. If you are the parent of a child with protruded teeth, please know that this is extremely common. In fact, I have never had a parent who brought their child in for treatment of severe protrusion not tell me that their child was being bullied because of it. That being said, it is so rewarding to see that same child blossom into a confident little boy or girl once their front teeth are brought back into place.

Extra or Missing Teeth

Having extra teeth, also called supernumerary teeth, doesn't automatically mean Phase 1 treatment is required. However, extra teeth can sometimes cause enough crowding to keep the regular teeth from growing in properly or even growing in at all. Sometimes the extra tooth itself becomes impacted and can later have a cyst form around it. Other times, the extra tooth grows into the mouth along with the other teeth and no one notices it because it just looks like the child has crowded teeth. In certain cases, though, especially in the case of a mesiodens (the name for an extra tooth that grows between the two upper front teeth), the eruption of an extra tooth can cause serious esthetic concerns that should be addressed sooner rather than later.

Treatment and management of an extra tooth or teeth can be as simple as having the extra tooth/teeth removed. Other times, however, it's more complex because the extra tooth has caused major displacement of the regular teeth. As with everything else, every case is unique and so these are treated on a case-by-case basis. If your dentist has told you that your child has an extra tooth, take your child for an orthodontic evaluation right away to see if the other teeth or their bite have been compromised in any way.

Missing teeth is a much different situation. Compared to extra teeth, missing teeth is much more common. Fortunately, the most common type of missing teeth are the wisdom teeth. However, this is followed by the lower second premolars and then by the upper lateral incisors (the teeth on each side of the upper two front teeth). In an x-ray, these will appear as one or more baby teeth with no permanent tooth underneath. If left alone, the baby teeth will typically stay in place until adulthood because there is no permanent tooth to push them out. Sometimes though, they do loosen and fall out, especially if a nearby permanent tooth was trying to come in. Overall, missing teeth do not cause the same problems of crowding and/or tooth impaction as do extra teeth. And while a child with missing teeth should be monitored, treatment of missing teeth typically happens later after the remaining permanent teeth have grown in and does not require Early (Phase 1) Treatment.

Eruption Problems

Sometimes the permanent teeth misbehave and don't erupt (grow in) where they are supposed to. Crowding is one reason for this but other times it is due to genetic factors we don't really understand. When my adult patient Kevin came in for a consultation, his chief complaint was a lower left canine tooth that had erupted on the tongue side of his lower jaw for no apparent reason. He was not crowded. I explained to Kevin that moving that large tooth from the inside of his lower jaw to its correct place would not be simple

The type of treatment required depends on which tooth is in question, as well as the severity of the tooth displacement.

and would take some time, along with some fancy orthodontic appliances. Kevin wanted his tooth in place so we started treatment. Several months after starting his own treatment, he trusted us enough to bring his daughter Eva in for an evaluation. Lo and behold, she had the same lower-left canine growing in on the inside of her lower jaw. Like father, like daughter. For Eva though, things were going to be a lot easier because she was not done growing and developing and we could intervene before her canine got out of place as much as Kevin's had.

The term for when a tooth is growing into the wrong place is *ectopic eruption*. Ectopic eruption occurs because the tooth bud develops in the wrong spot inside the jaws. While this is rare, it happens enough that every orthodontic office has several new patients each month that come in with ectopically erupting teeth. Ectopic eruption is most common with the upper first molars and the upper canines but can really happen with any tooth. With the canines—and especially the upper ones—ectopic eruption can lead to canine tooth impaction even in the absence of crowding. For teeth other than molars, ectopic eruption can lead to two "rows" of teeth: One row where the ectopic permanent teeth grew in and another row that has the baby teeth that didn't get pushed out.

The type of treatment required depends on which tooth is in question, as well as the severity of the tooth displacement. However, this is something that typically requires immediate intervention of some type to prevent longer and more complicated treatment later.

Appliances Commonly Used during Phase 1 Treatment

The appliances used during Phase 1 are as variable as the reasons for doing the treatment. Typically, braces are only placed on the permanent teeth, but because dentofacial orthopedics is often involved in Phase 1 treatment, there are myriad appliances that are used, as well. The next sections contain appliances commonly used in Phase 1 treatment.

RPE/Expander

The RPE, which stands for rapid palatal expander, is most often just called an "expander," but if you were to read through nerdy orthodontic books, you would discover that this appliance has tons of different names due to the many variations in its design.

Expanders are often used because the most common type of jaw growth problem is an upper jaw that is too narrow, and expanders widen the upper jaw of a growing child. Rapid palatal expander is itself a misnomer, since there is nothing rapid about the expansion process. The appliance, which typically hooks up to the first molars and first premolars, has a small screw mechanism in the center, which is turned by a little key. It sounds complex, but it's quite simple and we always teach parents how to do the turns with the key we give them. At our office, we even have a YouTube video that we text to parents that shows them how to turn the expander mechanism. The expansion is very gradual but you will see the wonderful effects right away.

Lower Expander

Some orthodontists recommend an expander for the lower jaw even though, as we have already learned, the lower jaw cannot be expanded. When an orthodontist recommends this appliance, please know that unlike the upper, the lower jaw itself is not truly being expanded (since it anatomically can't be), but rather it is the lower teeth that are being tipped out to widen the dental arch. There is certainly more than one way to do things, but I feel that dental arch widening can just as easily be accomplished with braces, so there is no reason to place an appliance that can cause tongue soreness and speech difficulties.

Headgear

When most people think of headgear, they think of movies like *Sixteen Candles* where the uber-nerdy kids wear headgear to school or outside the home. The Hollywood image is that of a socially outcast kid with bulky metal braces and wires that go around his face and keep him from being normal.

I keep seeing a trend of doctors advertising their practices to be "headgear free." I find this type of marketing a little concerning because I feel it is using the fear of headgear to promote their office.

A long time ago, kids did wear headgear to school. Not today, though. The requirement is twelve to fourteen hours per day at home, and this includes sleeping hours. So we are talking about eight hours during sleep and four to six hours at home, while awake.

I know that nobody dreams of wearing headgear and I rarely recommend it myself. However, in an era where orthodontic gadgets come and go, headgear is still around for one reason: it works and it works well. If your child has severe protrusion, especially if it is related to a protrusive upper jaw bone, headgear is still a great option. Thanks to advances in orthodontics such as TADs and modern functional appliances (I'll explain those later), the use of headgear has been greatly reduced. But every case is different, so if your orthodontists recommends it for your child, ask them why headgear and not the other options. They may have a good reason. If they don't give you a good reason, consider a second opinion.

I keep seeing a trend of doctors advertising their practices to be "headgear free." I find this type of marketing a little concerning because I feel it is using the fear of headgear to promote their office. I agree that, most of the time, there are better, more modern ways. But sometimes headgear is the best option. It just depends on the case and this doesn't necessarily make the orthodontist old-fashioned. In the last five years of seeing hundreds and hundreds of patients, I've recommended headgear fewer than ten times, and believe me, I've had more than ten patients with big overbites. One of those times it was on a young girl who couldn't wear a functional appliance (which causes the lower jaw to move forward) due to concerns about her TMJs which suffer from juvenile arthritis.

Facemask (Reverse-Pull Headgear)

Like regular headgear, facemask or reverse-pull headgear has also been around for a long time and works well, though it looks totally different. It also needs to be worn twelve to fourteen hours per day. Unlike regular headgear, which is used to correct overbites, however, the facemask is used to correct underbites and therefore works by "pulling" on the upper jaw of a growing child to help it grow forward. Because underbites are often the result of small upper jaws, facemask or reverse-pull headgears are often used in conjunction with expanders that widen the upper jaw.

This is important to note. The timing for using a facemask is critical, as it does not work well after a certain age. Remember when I said the bone joints around the upper jaw of children begin to fuse more and more as they get older and older? This is exactly why facemask works better (if not only) in young children. In many cases, successful facemask therapy can help patients avoid jaw surgery later in life.

Functional Appliances

Functional appliances are appliances that, like headgear, are designed to help correct large overbites. There are two main differences that distinguish the functional appliance from headgear. One is that functional appliances are worn exclusively inside the mouth. The other difference is that, unlike headgear, which works on the upper jaw, functional appliances work on the lower jaw, seeking to redirect and encourage its growth. And indeed, a small lower jaw is one of the main causes of large overbites. That being said, whether a functional appliance can actually grow the lower jaw has always been up for debate. Nevertheless, they do correct overbites, whether it grows the lower jaw or just tips the teeth.

While there are many removable styles of functional appliances, most of which look like retainers on steroids, it is the fixed (non-removable) functional appliances that have a big edge over headgear, because they do not rely on patient compliance.

Below is a list of common functional appliances, though be aware that there are many more.

Removable:
- Twin Block
- Bionator
- Frankel
- Swartz Double Plate

Fixed:
- Herbst
- Jasper Jumper
- Mara
- Forsus

Timing is Everything: Two Case Studies

Ben and Catherine

When Ben and Catherine's mom brought them to our office, it was really mainly for Ben. Ben was eleven years old, in middle school, and had crooked teeth. His little sister Catherine was seven, very tiny, and had to be the cutest little girl in three counties. Their family dentist had referred Ben to our office for orthodontic treatment, but mom thought she should have her younger daughter checked out as well. Ben did indeed have crooked teeth, especially on the lower, but he still had twelve baby teeth left. Furthermore, his jaws were developing normally and his x-rays showed no indication that his adult teeth would have trouble erupting into his mouth. Catherine, on the other hand, had a severely narrow upper jaw that had resulted in severe crowding and had already caused a crossbite between her back teeth on the left side. The crossbite wasn't a true crossbite but rather the result of a functional shift. Basically, when Catherine's jaws came together in their natural position, her back teeth could not meet because of her narrow upper jaw, so she would shift her jaw to the left to be able to close.

Ben was in middle school and Catherine was only seven. The result of the evaluations were that I placed Ben on our Pre-Orthodontic Guidance Program so that I could monitor him until he was ready for braces. He was eleven years old but he was still not ready. Catherine, on the other hand, I started with Phase 1 treatment right away, which included an expander to widen her upper jaw.

Catherine was lucky that she had a dentist who was looking out for her and a mom who thought to bring her in for an orthodontic consultation. However, every month I meet someone who wasn't that lucky, and even though they can still be corrected with surgery, it always breaks my heart a little, knowing the surgery might have been able to be avoided with early treatment.

Vanessa

Vanessa was fifteen years old when she came to my office. She had an anterior and a posterior crossbite. Basically, her entire upper jaw fit inside of the lower jaw. She had no functional shift and had a true skeletal crossbite, which meant her crossbites were due to the large size difference between her upper and lower jaws. After diagnosing her case, I advised her mom that I could improve the posterior crossbite, but only jaw surgery could correct Jennifer's underbite. Her mom asked me how much jaw surgery cost. I gave her a range.

She stayed quiet for one moment and then replied, "I cannot afford that. Can you at least straighten her teeth and she can get surgery when she's an adult if she wants?"

I told Mom that I certainly could straighten Jennifer's teeth and improve Jennifer's posterior crossbite but then asked her if she would at least consider seeing an oral surgeon for a consultation.

Mom looked me in the eye without saying anything at first and then said, "Doctor, I took a bus to come see you. I cannot afford surgery, but I can afford your payment plan."

Today, Vanessa is still my patient and she is almost done with her braces. Her posterior crossbite is improved and when she smiles she flashes pretty, straight teeth. However, she still has a large underbite. I encourage her to think about surgery when she's an adult. She says she will. Not long after she started treatment, I felt comfortable enough to ask Mom why she had not brought her to an orthodontist sooner. She said, "I was waiting for her baby teeth to fall out."

Chapter 6

FOR GROWN-UPS ONLY

"It's never too late to be what you might have been."
—George Eliot

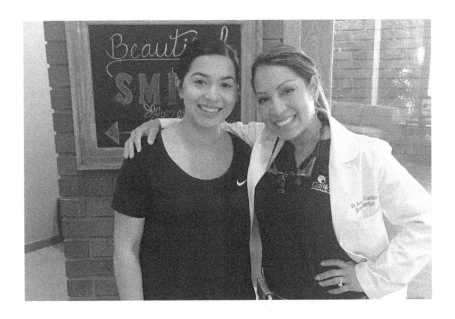

Noelle and her daughter Sarah came to our office to get beautiful straight teeth. They were hoping to get Invisalign, and they were hoping to start treatment together. The only problem was that Noelle, who was seventy-six years old, thought she wouldn't be able to get orthodontic treatment because of her osteoporosis.

It was December and a snow storm had just hit Salem, Oregon, yet Noelle came in with a fierce outfit which included an equally fierce white fur hat. She was sassy and full of energy. I thought to myself, "I'll definitely call your doctor, but I doubt anything can ever stop you from getting

It is never too late.

what you want." After calling her physician, I was happy to inform Noelle that she was clear for orthodontic treatment and could start whenever she and Sarah were ready. From the beginning, it was a joy to have them in our office and it was so cute how mother and daughter did everything together. Indeed, they acted more like sisters. Noelle finished her Invisalign treatment ahead of schedule and is now rocking beautiful straight teeth. It is never too late.

Noelle may be an extreme example and indeed most of the adult orthodontic patients in our office are much younger than that; the average age is probably more like thirty-five. The point is, I believe that orthodontics should be approached like anything else in life. Time will pass no matter what. The only difference is that you either accomplish your goals by the end of that time, or you do not. When I decided to go to dental school, I was twenty-five years old and, like many twenty-five-year-olds, I was delusional and thought I was old. It dawned on me that if I attended dental school, I would be almost thirty by the time I got out. I mean, that would make me like a dinosaur, right? During that time, a really close friend of mine told me, "Ana, you're going to be thirty years old one day no matter what. The only difference is that if you go to dental school, you'll be a doctor and if you don't, then you won't." That stuck with me ever since and it has been how I've approached most long-term goals in my life.

A beautiful, confident smile is no different. Having braces as an adult for twelve to twenty-four months may seem like an eternity but the time will pass anyway. Think how many times you have said to yourself, "Wow, it's April already? I feel like Christmas just ended." I know I say things like that all the time. And like I said, the time will pass anyway; except that at the end of those twenty months you will have a beautiful smile and healthy bite if you proceeded with orthodontics, or you will just have your current smile if you didn't. You decide.

Are Adult Braces Cool Now?

The answer is, quite simply, yes, adult braces are cool. No, I'm not the only one that thinks so. As I mentioned in Chapter 3, adults are seeking and getting orthodontic treatment in record numbers. A 2014 survey titled "Economics of Orthodontics" by the American Association of Orthodontics (AAO) estimates that at least 27 percent of orthodontic patients in the US and Canada are adults. When I first started my office, it was 15 percent adults, on a good day. However, our adult patient population has steadily increased year after year and is now over 37 percent and still increasing.

We live in a world where personal image is critically important, both to external success and to a person's impression of themselves. A powerful self-image works to help improve somebody's self-confidence. Improving self-confidence can lead to greater opportunity for an individual. More and more adults are finding that having crooked teeth and a bad bite can be a hindrance to confidence and can negatively impact potential success. Not to mention that few things will

The staff is so kind and patient with my daughter (she has a lot of anxiety). We moved to Portland shortly after we started with Dr. Castilla, but we are sticking with her because the quality of care is well worth the drive!

—*Lindsie P.*

make you look older than crooked teeth worn down by a bad bite. In the past, not only was there a stigma associated with adult orthodontics, but it was also more complicated because the technology needed to address the unique needs of adult orthodontic treatment was simply not there. Therefore, many adults would simply live with their crooked teeth.

We live in a world where personal image is critically important, both to external success and to a person's impression of themselves.

But not anymore. According to the AAO, the number of adult patients seen by orthodontists increased by 14 percent between 2010 and 2012, reaching 1.2 million adults. By 2014, that figure jumped another 16 percent to, 1.4 million. This study also found that more men are opting for orthodontic treatment. As of 2012, 44 percent of adult patients were male, compared to 29 percent in 2010.[8]

Not Your Daughter's Orthodontics

If you are an adult considering orthodontic treatment, it is important to understand that there are some things that make adult orthodontic treatment unique. These things sometime require a multi-disciplinary approach which means your orthodontist will have to work closely with your dentist, periodontist, oral surgeon, or other dental specialist. Below are some of the top things you should definitely know about if you are an adult considering orthodontic treatment.

---

8   AAO, "A Study to Smile About."

Adults Are Done Growing

One of the major differences between adult and child orthodontic treatment is that adults are done growing. For this reason, orthopedic treatment to guide the development of the jaws cannot be performed on adults. If the bad bite or malocclusion is severe, orthognathic (jaw) surgery may be needed to correct the bite. Think of the example I gave in the last chapter on early treatment where a child can have their upper jaw bone widened with an appliance called an expander, but an adult can only accomplish this with jaw surgery.

It's Important to Have Healthy Gums

Another consideration is the health of your gums. Unfortunately, 47 percent of all adults age thirty and over have periodontal disease, which is also known as gum disease. This number jumps to a staggering 70 percent for adults sixty-five years of age and over.[9] Periodontal disease is the process by which the tissues surrounding the roots of the teeth (i.e., the bone and gums), slowly but surely deteriorate and become lost due to chronic inflammation caused by the bacteria present in dental plaque and tartar. Because orthodontic treatment moves your teeth through your jaw bones, it is critical that your gums are healthy and that you are not among the 47 percent of adults with periodontal disease. Periodontal disease causes bone loss, and how can you safely move teeth that don't have that much bone around them?

Whether you are considering orthodontic treatment or not, it is important that you see your dentist to make sure you don't have periodontal disease. That being said, just because you have a history

---

9   P. I. Eke et al., "Prevalence of Periodontitis in Adults in the United States: 2009 and 2010," *J Dent Res* 91: 914–920.

of periodontal disease doesn't mean you are not a candidate for braces. Many times, if the disease process has been arrested by your dentist, you can still proceed with orthodontic treatment as long as it remains under control. If you've had periodontal disease in the past or suspect you might have it now, check with your primary care dentist to make sure it is safe for you to proceed with orthodontics.

Unfortunately, 47 percent of all adults age thirty and over have periodontal disease, which is also known as gum disease. This number jumps to a staggering 70 percent for adults sixty-five years of age and over.

Think Twice Before Spending Major Bucks on Dental Work

If you have unfortunately lost one or more of your permanent teeth and are now wearing prosthetic replacements such as dental bridges and implants, please know that these cannot be moved by braces. It definitely doesn't mean that you cannot benefit from orthodontic treatment. It simply means that all your other teeth will move, but your dental implant and bridge will not. Let me give you an example. Let's say you lost a molar when you were young and didn't have much money to get it fixed. You're now older and have a job with dental insurance and want to get a dental implant to replace it. Before you get that implant, take a good look in the mirror and ask yourself if you will ever want to get your teeth straightened or your bite fixed. If you are uncertain if your bite would benefit from correction, then you should see an orthodontist for a consultation first. I say this because, once your dental implant is in, you will not be able to correct your bite orthodontically, unless the correction is very minor. This is because the implant cannot be moved with braces (or Invisalign). It is fused to your jaw bone. Truly it is a domino effect since the immobility of even one implant can limit the movement of the surrounding natural teeth.

So if you have an overbite that requires braces with rubber bands to fix (to move the upper teeth back) but you have an upper bridge or implant, then your upper teeth on the side of the bridge or implant won't be able to move back for correction of the overbite. I can't tell you how many times I have had an adult patient come to me and say, "Dr. Castilla, I just got all my cavities fixed and my missing teeth replaced last month. I got a clean bill of dental health and now I'm ready for braces." Sigh. This is the part when I have to break it to them that I can't fix their overbite because their implants won't move.

The moral of the story is, please see an orthodontist before spending money on an implant or bridge. You may find that due to your type of bite, it is best to correct it with orthodontic treatment first and then get the implant at the end of your braces. Or even better: You may discover that you don't need that implant after all. This is especially true in cases of recent tooth loss, where an orthodontist may simply be able to close the space left behind by the tooth extraction.

What about other dental work? While fillings don't really affect the movement of teeth, they should ideally be done before orthodontic treatment is started. Crowns (sometimes known as caps), on the other hand, are a little bit different. Because a crown changes the entire shape of your tooth, it is best if they are done after completion of your orthodontic treatment. What I mean is, when a crown is made, it is shaped so that it fits well with the surrounding teeth as well as with the teeth on the opposing jaw. That's all wonderful when your bite is good. But what if it's not? That just means that when you get braces later and fix your bite, your crown may not fit with the opposing teeth in the new, corrected bite. That is, the crown was shaped to fit to your old bite, not your new bite. This problem is often a bigger issue with crowns that were made for anterior teeth before orthodontic treatment. When the crown is made, it's made to fit in a reduced space along with all the other crooked front teeth. The teeth then get straightened and now it is clear that the crown on one of your front teeth is skinnier than the crown on the other front tooth. Thus, it is not uncommon for adult patients to need some of their crown work remade after completing orthodontic treatment.

So what should you do if your dentist says you have a big cavity on one of your molars and it will need a crown? Are you really going to wait eighteen months for your orthodontic treatment to be complete and let your cavity grow bigger and bigger during that time? Absolutely not! You can ask your dentist to give you a large filling temporarily or, if this is not possible, ask him or her to give you a temporary crown that you can wear while you are in orthodontic treatment. When

> *Thus, it is not uncommon for adult patients to need some of their crown work remade after completing orthodontic treatment.*

you complete your orthodontic treatment and your bite is corrected, then you can then go back to your dentist to get it replaced with a much stronger final or "permanent" crown.

Finally, though there have been improvements made in the bonding of braces or aligner attachments to porcelain and gold crowns, bond strength is still strongest to natural tooth enamel. Therefore, you may have to be extra careful with the foods you eat during orthodontic treatment if you have a lot of dental crowns.

When a Bad Bite Beats Up Your Teeth

Crooked teeth that are in malocclusion (bad bite) are not considered attractive. We all know that. But what many people don't realize is that a bad bite results in accelerated and premature tooth wear due to years of "clashing" of the teeth during speaking and chewing. This "clashing" or "banging" between the teeth occurs because the teeth are not in their correct positions. Thus, if you've reached middle age with a bad bite, chances are most of your teeth have suffered from moderate to severe wear. The wear, unfortunately, tends to be uneven and many times it is not readily evident to the patient before starting treatment. That is, when your teeth are crooked or crowded, it is difficult to tell that some of your teeth may be severely or unevenly worn or even cracked. All you see is the crowding. When your teeth become straight, it becomes readily apparent that one of your teeth is longer or not as worn as the other. If the wear is small, the orthodontist can do some enameloplasty or re-shaping of the teeth to even them out. If the wear is of a larger magnitude, you may need tooth-colored fillings, veneers, or even crowns to restore the shape of the teeth after your orthodontic treatment is complete. When visiting an orthodontist for a treatment consultation, make sure to ask about this if you've lived with crowding or a bad bite for a long time.

I Lost My Tooth. Now What?

As I explained, if you have lost a tooth recently, I highly recommend you see an orthodontist before getting any type of prosthetic replacement. If it's been a while since the tooth loss happened, ask the orthodontist if the space can still be closed. In general, if the tooth loss happened within five years, the space can be closed but not if it's been longer than that, due to the bone loss that occurs after losing a tooth. Also, ask if any orthodontic auxiliaries or supplemental treatments will be needed, since space closure in adults is more challenging. Often times, the closing of a space may require temporary anchorage devices (TADs) or accelerating treatments, such as Propel. I will discuss these options, along with other treatments unique to adults.

Temporary Anchorage Devices (TADs)

No discussion of adult orthodontic treatment would be complete without at least a mention of Temporary Anchorage Devices (TADs), also called mini-implants. However, these are not to be confused with dental implants that are used to replace missing teeth, though like dental implants, TADs are made of medical quality, biocompatible titanium alloy.

So what is a TAD? A TAD is a miniature screw that is placed in the jaw bone to provide your orthodontist with a stable anchorage — that is, a fixed point around which, typically, other teeth can be moved. TADs can be placed in a variety of places inside the mouth but are most commonly placed in the roof of the mouth or between the roots of certain teeth.

The advent of TADs has made it possible for orthodontist to perform complex tooth movements or treat severe malocclusions (bad bites) that previously only surgery or headgear could accomplish. And though it sounds majorly invasive, placing a TAD is actually relatively simple for the doctor that is trained to do it, as it is for the patient receiving the TAD. Placement of a TAD is a minimally invasive procedure with virtually no recovery time. After the area where the TAD will be placed is numbed with an injection or other numbing treatment, a patient feels only gentle pressure as the TAD is inserted. The whole process can take just minutes to complete. Afterward, an over-the-counter pain reliever can be taken if needed—but many patients need no pain reliever at all. Taking TADs out is even easier. This is because, unlike dental implants which fuse to the bone, TADs do not fuse to your jawbone and are simply mechanically retained. I have placed many TADs and so I can confidently tell you that it is nowhere near as invasive as my patients imagined when I first told them about it. In fact, many patients have actually told me afterward, "Wow, that was a lot easier than I thought."

The advent of TADs has made it possible for orthodontist to perform complex tooth movements or treat severe malocclusions (bad bites) that previously only surgery or headgear could accomplish.

Let me give you an example. Let's say someone has what is called a skeletal open bite. A skeletal open bite is often caused when the back side of the upper jaw is "too tall" or "too long" in an up-and-down direction. This causes the lower jaw to wedge open, which in turn results in an open bite between the front teeth, so the front teeth don't meet. It's simply a matter of genetics. Some people are born with upper jaws that are too tall. In the past, the only option for a good, stable result would have been a surgery that required the back of the upper jaw to be surgically intruded or pulled up. Now, a TAD can be placed in the roof of the mouth (not as painful as it sounds) and the upper molars can instead be pushed into the upper jaw by pulling on them from the TAD in the roof of the mouth. After the upper molars have been pushed (or intruded) into the upper jaw, the lower jaw can close down some more and the open bite between the front teeth is corrected. This is just one of many examples of the type of treatment that braces in combination with TADs can accomplish. Other examples include reduction of severely large overbites and closure of a tooth space after the tooth has been lost or removed.

There are many TAD systems out there, but the really important question for you to ask if your or your teen's orthodontic treatment plan includes TADs, is this: Is the orthodontist placing your TAD(s)? Some orthodontists place TADs, but most of them don't, so you will have to be referred to an oral surgeon to get this done. This is perfectly fine, of course, but you may want to ask what surgeon you will be referred to.

I mentioned this question in Chapter 3 but I think it's worth repeating. If your or your teen's treatment plan requires TADs, make sure to ask about extra fees. If the orthodontist is referring you to an outside doctor (such as an oral surgeon) for TAD placement, then there will obviously be a separate fee, but if the orthodontist himself is placing the TAD, ask if the quoted fee for treatment includes the TAD placement or if you will get charged a separate fee later. And, of course, you'll want to know the amount of the fee.

Treatment Accelerators

Today's orthodontic technology allows for treatment that is more comfortable and also faster than ever before. Nevertheless, some patients desire even faster treatment options. Accordingly, the science of treatment acceleration is rapidly evolving and there are now more options for those that want ultra-fast orthodontic treatment.

Be aware, however, that there will be an increase in your treatment fee with all these methods. For some methods, it is a small increase whereas for other methods, the increase in fee is significant. This is something to consider if the cost of treatment is a major concern for you. Here is a list of some of the current options available in treatment acceleration:

MECHANICAL PULSATION DEVICES

These devices are probably the most popular form of treatment acceleration due to their relatively low cost (average cost is about $1,100 in addition to the orthodontic treatment fees) and non-invasiveness. Basically, they are vibrating mouthpieces that you bite on for twenty minutes a day. The idea is that the low-frequency mechanical pulsation increases the cellular activity that is already taking place during orthodontic treatment in the bone surrounding your teeth. Thus, bone remodels at a faster rate and your teeth can move faster as well. As a bonus, some clinical studies (and many patients) claim that the pulsations decrease discomfort associated with orthodontic tooth movement. The device most commonly associated with this technology is AcceleDent, who currently claims that treatment time with the use of their device can be reduced by as much as 50 percent.

CORTICOTOMY

Corticotomy refers to the process of making cuts on the outer part of bone, called the cortex. It is used to speed up orthodontic treatment by creating an influx of healing cells that cause a lot of bone cell turnover. In orthodontics, teeth are able to move through the jaw bone precisely due to the bone cell turnover that is created by the pressure of the braces. With corticotomy, this turnover is increased and, therefore, the tooth movement is able to speed up. Of all the tooth accelerating procedures, corticotomy has been around the longest, is the most researched, and creates the fastest tooth movement. The major disadvantages are that is it the most expensive and also the most invasive.

Below is a list of different corticotomy procedures:

- **Wilckodontics** (also known as Accelerated Osteogenic Orthodontics). This is the most invasive and expensive, but also the fastest.

- **Piezocision.** Not as invasive as Wilckodontics, since it does not require stitches or bone grafting. It is also less expensive.

- **Micro-osteoperforation (MOP).** This procedure was made popular by the Propel Orthodontics device, which creates small perforations in the bone around the teeth, creating the acceleration of tooth movement, as described above. This is the least invasive of the corticotomy procedures and can, therefore, be performed by an orthodontist.

PHOTOBIOMODULATION (PBM)

While this sounds intense, photobiomodulation consists of simple device that uses low-energy-level light pulses to stimulate the bone and gum tissues surrounding the roots of your teeth and increase bone cell turnover. This, as we have learned, facilitates tooth movement. The device, which is called OrthoPulse, is placed inside your mouth and it looks very similar to the mechanical pulsation devices, except it uses light instead of vibration.

If you are considering a treatment-accelerating procedure, especially if it is one of the corticotomies, it is important that you select a provider that is well trained in the management of accelerated orthodontic treatment. Also, please don't confuse accelerated treatment, which uses the latest technology under the care of a specialist to speed up comprehensive treatment that gives you beautiful straight teeth and a healthy bite, with cosmetic improvement-only treatments that are provided by some general dentists, which usually only correct the alignment of your front teeth and not your bite. These are totally different things.

> *Of all the tooth accelerating procedures, corticotomy has been around the longest, is the most researched, and creates the fastest tooth movement.*

Limited treatment

Most adult patients will benefit best from comprehensive orthodontic treatment to correct not just the misalignment of their teeth, but to also obtain a healthy bite. However, since the goal of comprehensive orthodontic treatment is to establish an ideal bite, this type of treatment may not fit the unique goals you have for your smile.

Perhaps you already had orthodontic treatment and have minor relapse of a couple of front teeth. Or maybe your primary care dentist needs a tooth uprighted to create a better space for a dental implant. Depending on your particular case and your particular smile goals, there are some instances where limited orthodontic treatment may be appropriate.

Limited treatment usually involves braces or Invisalign in one of the two dental arches. That is, the braces or aligners go on either upper teeth only or lower teeth only, depending on the case and smile goals of the person. This is usually done when the bite in the back is good but there are some minor rotations of the front teeth or small spaces between them. Other times, limited treatment is not done to fix the bite but to accommodate dental work.

Because this type of treatment is limited in nature, treatment times are shorter, with most cases finishing in six to ten months.

As you can see, though adult orthodontic treatment is more popular than ever, there is a lot more than meets the eye here. I received treatment as an adult and it changed my life. I believe it can do the same for you. However, there are a lot of things to consider if you are an adult looking to get braces, so it is important to do your homework. My hope is that you can use this information to help you ask the right questions when looking for an orthodontist.

Chapter 7

YOUR SMILE INVESTMENT

"Price is what you pay. Value is what you get."
Warren Buffet

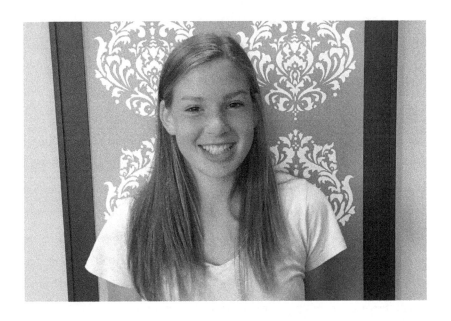

Making orthodontic treatment afford-able—not cheap—is a subject that I am very passion-ate about. I didn't get braces until I got a job after college, specifically because my parents could not afford to get them for me when I was a kid. I understand that it is a large investment and that it can even

seem too expensive. Investing in orthodontic treatment for yourself or your child is one of those lifetime investments. After all, we're talking about the smile of your life here. Every time you smile at your children, every time you smile at your spouse, every time you smile during a job interview, you only have one smile to give. We smile during the best moments of our life. This is an investment not only in your health but also in your self-confidence and in your future.

The truth is that the cost of orthodontic treatment has actually not increased relative to inflation over time. In fact, the opposite is true. The cost of braces has actually declined on an inflation-adjusted basis over the past fifty years. In the 1960s, braces cost $2,000. That would be about $16,000 today when you adjust for inflation. The main reason for this is that advances in orthodontic technology have allowed for faster, more efficient treatment that requires fewer visits. This is great news, not only for you as a patient, but also for orthodontists who can now help more people because more people can afford it.

My goal in writing this chapter is not to sell you on the value of orthodontic treatment or a beautiful smile. That sells itself. My goal is to provide enough information for you to make a great financial investment and feel confident that you can afford a beautiful smile for yourself or a loved one. This is truer now than at any other time in the history of braces. From extended financing to health insurance to paying with pre-tax dollars, there are several things you should consider prior to paying for orthodontic treatment.

Flexible Financing

Every orthodontic office has a different philosophy about this and, therefore, you will find that payment plans vary greatly at different offices. We already know that orthodontic treatment is an important investment and that finding the right doctor and office is critical. But if affordability is important to you, then it is important that you ask about flexible financing.

Most practices offer zero-interest in-house financing, but not all of them are equally flexible in their payment plans. Typically, the payment plan requires a down payment, with the rest of the cost financed over the length of the treatment. So, for example, if your treatment is estimated at eighteen months, then you pay for your treatment via a combination of a down payment with the remaining balance split over eighteen months. If you need lower monthly payments, then your options are either to pay a higher down payment or to get extended financing. Extended financing refers to payment plans that allow you to pay the cost of treatment beyond your estimated treatment time, thus lowering your monthly payment. In our example above, instead of paying your balance over eighteen months, you would pay it over twenty-four or more months.

If extended financing is offered to you, make sure you are clear about any interest rates that may apply for extending the payment plan. At our office, we offer both low down payments and extended financing, all at zero interest. Thanks to our flexible financing, we have had families who were able to afford two or even three kids in treatment all at the same time.

Insurance

First of all, I want to emphatically state that you do not need orthodontic insurance in order to afford orthodontic treatment for you and your family. In fact, more than half of patients seeking orthodontic treatment do not have orthodontic insurance coverage. But if you do, congrats. I have some tips for you to consider. I'm no insurance expert, so the information here is not to be taken as insurance advice.

Love Dr. Castilla and all of her fun-loving staff. We always feel welcome and well-cared for beyond just the braces! They really care about each patient.

—*Lisa H.*

But over the years, I have learned more than I ever wanted to know about this dry, but so important, topic.

All insurance plans are different, so it's important to be your own advocate in terms of understanding the benefits of your insurance plan. Just because your employer says you have coverage for braces doesn't mean you are fully covered—or even covered at all. In fact, in our area, the range of coverage is between $1,000 and $3,000, with an average of $1,500. Additionally, there can be age limitations. When I was ready to get braces for myself, I was told by the HR department at my job that my dental health insurance plan covered orthodontics. However, later I found out this coverage was only until age nineteen. Since I was already older than that, I had to pay for the entire cost out of pocket.

Another thing to know is that pretty much every single insurance that covers you for orthodontic treatment will only offer you a one-time benefit. That is, if your plan has $1,500 of coverage, that is a one-time event. It is not like your general dentistry benefit that renews each year. You get that $1,500 one time. Ever.

If you and your spouse or another household family member have separate dental health insurance plans, then it is possible that you can get coverage from your insurance and from your family member's insurance on top of that. This is called *dual coverage* and most insurance companies we've worked with do allow this. However, be aware that it is not always allowed. For example, if you and your spouse each have separate orthodontic insurance benefits from different employers and you file insurance with your insurance first and then try to file for coverage with your spouse's insurance, your spouse's insurance company may not pay out because you've already been covered by your insurance. If you or your child is covered by two or more insurance plans, it is important that your insurance companies conduct what's called a "Coordination of Benefits" so that you know exactly how these insurance plans can work together.

Exactly how your insurance pays is also very important. Some insurance plans pay the entire benefit at once. That is, if you have a benefit of $1,000, then $1,000 is paid out when the claim is filed. Other plans pay the benefit on a payment schedule, such as a monthly or quarterly basis. What this means for you is that if your plan pays in installments, and for some reason you drop your insurance coverage the following year and they haven't finished paying your benefit, they likely will not finish paying and you won't receive your full benefit. The same goes if you stop working at your current job before the insurance company is done paying.

> *Health insurance can be very complex, especially because each plan is so different and there are so many variations and nuances by state or region.*

Health insurance can be very complex, especially because each plan is so different and there are so many variations and nuances by state or region. The best thing is to be your own advocate and ask all the questions you need to ask so that you are fully informed. Additionally, most orthodontists will provide you with a complimentary insurance check so you are not alone in figuring it out.

Flexible Spending Accounts (FSAs) and
Health Savings Accounts (HSAs)

Many employers offer FSAs or HSAs to their employees as a benefit to help their employees manage their health expenses throughout the year. The differences between these two types of accounts is beyond the scope of this book, so for now let's just say that they're both accounts to which you can contribute tax-free dollars for payment of qualified medical expenses, such as orthodontics. If you are considering orthodontic treatment for yourself or for a family member, it would be good to inquire if your employer offers either of these types of accounts, since this is one of the best ways to save on orthodontic treatment.

There are a couple of things to note if you are considering the use of an FSA or HSA. HSA allows for higher balances than an FSA, so if you have an HSA, this means that you may be able to pay for your entire orthodontic treatment tax-free. However, you do have to qualify for an HSA, so ask your company's HR department for the rules. For an FSA, there are no requirements to qualify but the maximum you can save is lower. There are other differences too. Unlike an HSA, whose balance can be carried over from year to year, the funds in an FSA account must be used by the end of the year or you lose them.

If you have an FSA, there are a couple of other things to know. One is that you should make sure that you are aware of your employer's enrollment period, because if you miss it, then you will have to wait until the next enrollment period to get your FSA money. Once you know when the enrollment period is, you need to know how much you want to contribute to your FSA for your orthodontic treatment, since it is required that you tell them ahead of time.

Meaning, you can't tell them you want to save $1,000 and then later say, "I really want to save $2,000." Therefore, you'll want to see an orthodontist for a consultation prior to your FSA enrollment period so that you know how much money you will need to save. Fortunately, most orthodontist offices offer free consultations.

Third-Party Financing Companies (Medical Credit Cards)

Patients will sometimes ask us about using medical credit cards, such as Care Credit, to finance their orthodontic treatment. In my mind, there is no doubt that you can find an orthodontic office that will work with you on creating a customized, flexible payment plan that will suit your family budget, so I usually discourage patients from using these types of third-party financing companies unless absolutely necessary. The problem is that many of these medical credit cards offer financing deals that are typically accompanied by a dangerous deferred interest feature. When this deferred interest does kick in, the interest rates can be really high—as high as 28 percent! If you do decide to go with this option, make sure you read all the fine print so you are not trapped by a crazy-high interest rate.

Choose a Skilled Orthodontist and a High-Quality Office

If you are concerned about cost, you might be tempted to go with the cheapest office, even if they are not the most skilled or experienced. But by cutting corners now you may be putting yourself at risk for future complications. You only want to do braces once in your life and you don't want to end up with complications or damage caused by improper treatment. So get it done right the first time. Otherwise, you may end up paying much more than the initial cost of braces when all is said and done.

Also, be careful of hidden fees or tricky fee presentations. I once saw a fee presentation from an orthodontic office where the "treatment fee" looked lower than average, but that fee did not include the required down payment or the fact that they were also requiring a records fee, which is a fee charged for the X-rays and photos. By the time you added the down payment and records fee, their fee was actually an average fee—but the payment plan required a large down payment. The way it was written, it looked like a great deal, but when you added all the other fees, it wasn't.

When fees are presented, make sure you ask questions about what is required to pay upfront and what the true total fee is. As discussed in Chapter 3, ask about additional fees for "esthetic" braces or auxiliary appliances, such as TADs. When comparing offices, you should especially look closely at the cheapest ones. This is because these offices often don't have an all-inclusive fee and charge for additional things such as retainers or missed appointments. Some so-called "lower priced" offices charge a monthly fee for every month that treatment extends past the estimated treatment time, even if you are done paying for the original treatment fee.

If you decide to go with Invisalign or other clear aligner treatment, make sure you ask about refinements. Refinements refer to additional aligners you get after you complete your first set of aligners. Basically, when your treatment plan is created, your orthodontist will give you a certain number of aligners that in theory should complete your case. This first set of aligners hardly ever accomplishes all the correction you need. Thus, you will need another set of aligners, called refinement aligners. Sometimes you even need a third or fourth set, depending on the complexity of your case. This is all a normal part of aligner treatment, but you want to make sure that these refinement aligners are included in your quoted fee and that there will not be any additional charge to obtain them later.

I believe everyone deserves a beautiful smile and that is why, at our office, we will not let finances get in the way of starting treatment.

I believe everyone deserves a beautiful smile and that is why, at our office, we will not let finances get in the way of starting treatment. Our goal is to create solutions, not obstacles, for our patients. We think of ourselves as "Smile Facilitators." I know that there are other orthodontists out there that feel the same way. I hope this chapter gave you some good information, and that you are confident in knowing that you can get the smile of your dreams, regardless of your budget.

Chapter 8

LIVING WITH YOUR SMILE UNDER CONSTRUCTION

"The art of life is a constant readjustment to our surroundings."
Kakuzo Okakura

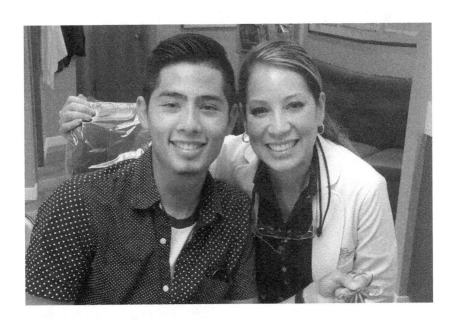

When I was a resident at Oregon Health and Science University, I had a young patient named Gina who I treated for Phase 1 orthodontic treatment. Despite being the most independent nine-year-old girl I have ever met (and I've met some trail blazers), Gina was amazing at following all the rules I gave her about her braces. The day she came to get them off, she marched into the clinic with the determination of a warrior and, before she ever made it to the dental chair, she pulled a bag of microwaveable popcorn out of her purse and exclaimed, "Where is your microwave?"

Aside from living without popcorn, you will find that living with braces is not anywhere near as difficult as you might imagine. Today's modern braces have made orthodontic treatment more comfortable than ever before, so don't let this concern keep you from getting the smile you've always wanted. When you first get braces there will definitely be an adjustment period. After all, we can't expect that wearing braces will feel the same as not wearing braces. Fortunately, this adjustment period is short. Everyone is different, of course, but for most people we are talking about three to seven days.

Beyond the adjustment period, you will have to make some temporary lifestyle changes. But most of these changes are small and will become second nature in short order. Those changes depend on the type of treatment you get, but they may involve many of the following.

Eating

The first day you get braces or clear aligners, there will be no discomfort. It will just feel weird. There's no other way to describe it. Kids, I think, have the best reaction to weird. One of my favorite things that happens in my office is the look on a little kid's face when the cheek retractors are removed and they first feel their braces against their lips. Most of the kids cannot stop giggling at how "weird" they think it feels. Some even say it "tickles." I always take this as a powerful lesson that it is we, as individuals, who assign meaning to everything in life. Weird can be uncomfortable or weird can be flat-out hilarious. You decide.

The day after you get braces is another thing. Here again, children often handle it better than adults, but either way, know that between days two and four you may feel sensitivity to pressure or "biting down." Thus, be sure to stick to soft foods for the first few days after getting braces. To this I say, "Yay! Bring on the pasta!" (And if you're old enough, the wine. Wine is also a soft food.)

After the initial adjustment period, you still have to be careful what you eat. Not because you'll be sore, but because you don't want your braces to break. That means avoiding overly crunchy or sticky foods, such as hard breads, raw vegetables, popcorn, nuts, and candy. Additionally, you will need to get rid of some questionable habits, such as chewing on pencils or pens and biting your fingernails. These habits not only cause damage to your braces, but they are also bad for your actual teeth. Often times, patients ask me if they will have to give up eating apples and carrots. The answer is, no you don't. But you do have to break them up into small pieces and stick them in the back of your mouth. Certainly, you can imagine that if you sink your front teeth into a whole apple, a couple of brackets might fly off into the distance.

If this all sounds very limiting, don't worry. You can still eat mostly everything. Braces don't stop any of my patients from enjoying a good, juicy burger. Or pizza. Besides, many of the foods you should avoid with braces are foods you should probably be avoiding anyway, like hard candy, caramel, etc.

If you've opted for Invisalign, you will not be limited in the foods that you eat. In fact, this is one of the major advantages of Invisalign. There is one thing you will have to give up though, or at least seriously limit. That one thing is snacking. I wore Invisalign

Dr. Castilla is a kind, thorough orthodontist who takes time to answer all your questions and explains everything too! The staff is friendly and professional. Great experiences with two of my kids so far!

—*Melissa H.*

for about five months last year to fix some very minor rotations, and the one thing I was surprised to learn about myself is how much I actually snacked. I had to nip that habit in the bud really quickly. The reason you have to give up or seriously limit snacking with Invisalign is that you have to wear them twenty-two hours per day. This gives you only two hours to eat and brush your teeth. And unless you are a vacuum cleaner of an eater, this is not a lot of time.

General Soreness

If you do experience any major discomfort, you can take an over-the-counter pain medication such as Tylenol or Advil. This will almost certainly take care of any pain while you are adjusting.

For sore or irritated lips, cheeks, and tongue, you can do a couple of things. If you are wearing fixed braces, simply apply dental wax over the offending bracket. This will serve to cushion the bracket against your lip or cheek. Most orthodontists will provide you with a sample of dental wax, but if you run out, you can find it in the dental aisle of just about any drug store or supermarket. Wax can be tricky to apply, though. A lot of people apply it only to find it falls off. The trick is to make sure the bracket is dry of any saliva. Wax will not stick to a wet bracket. How to dry your bracket? Use a Q-tip! Additionally, you have to press the wax over your bracket only once. If you over-manipulate the wax, it will start sticking to your finger instead of the bracket. Slap it on and move on.

With Invisalign, there are no wires or brackets to make your lips sore. But you will find that the attachments may initially feel rough against your lips and cheeks when you are eating and not wearing your aligners. This will go away with time and, at any rate, you will be wearing your aligners the vast majority of the time. One much more common source of initial discomfort with Invisalign is a feeling of "sharpness" along the edges of the aligners. This is particularly true on the tongue side of the aligners. Not because the aligner edges are truly sharper on the tongue side, but because when you first start wearing aligners, your tongue discovers a new "toy" to play with and be curious about. Eventually, you will stop constantly running your tongue along the edges of the aligners and this discomfort will go away. If you truly feel that you have a sharp edge somewhere, you can simply purchase a fine-grit nail file such as an emery board and smooth it away.

> *With Invisalign, there are no wires or brackets to make your lips sore.*

Cleaning Your Teeth

My favorite subject. I can't stress enough how important it is to keep your teeth clean—with or without braces. But I will speak more on that subject in the following chapter. For now, just know that when you're wearing braces, brushing and flossing will take longer than before. You may even need some extra tools, such as floss threaders, interproximal brushes (the little tiny brushes that look like miniature, white Christmas trees), or an oral irrigator, such as a WaterPik. Your orthodontist will give you instructions on how to brush and floss your teeth so you will have all the knowledge you need.

I always tell my patients that cleaning your teeth with braces is not difficult. And it really isn't. It's just more time consuming. Thus, the important thing is to help yourself by developing the habit of setting extra time after meals, and especially at the end of each day, for cleaning your teeth so that you can set yourself up for success. The last thing you want to do is stay in the habit of waiting till you're dead tired before getting ready for bed. You're definitely not going to want to spend time cleaning your teeth then.

Aside from this, it is even more important that you continue to visit your primary care dentist for professional cleanings and checkups. Unfortunately, most insurance plans cover cleanings only once or twice a year. I wish they could make an exception for patients in braces and let them get cleanings three times a year. That's how important it is to keep your teeth clean when you are in braces.

If you are an Invisalign patient, brushing and flossing will go a lot quicker, because you don't have to work around wires. But it is still not entirely a free ride. Many of your teeth will have attachments, and you still have to take extra care to clean around them.

For Invisalign and Clear Aligner Patients Only

Life with Invisalign or other clear aligners can be different from patients who have fixed braces. Below is a list of things that may give you an idea about what it's like to wear clear aligners:

- If you are a lady who is considering Invisalign, let me be the first one to tell you that you will get lipstick on your aligners. I discovered this early on in my Invisalign treatment. So if you're going to get dolled up, consider using a wear-resistant lip color, such as LipSense.

- As I've mentioned on multiple occasions, one of the huge benefits of wearing Invisalign or clear aligners is that it will be a lot quicker and even easier to clean your teeth. However, one thing that a lot of people never talk about is the fact that the aligners themselves stain and need to be cleaned. So, cleaning your teeth will be easier, but you also have to clean your aligners. Overall, the staining of aligners is not a huge deal, since you change to a new aligner every week. But even if you are careful to not drink colored drinks while wearing them and you brush them every night, by day five, they are slightly stained or "cloudy" and not as crystal-clear as in day one. I used to recommend cleaning them with soapy water or white vinegar, but since then, I have discovered an aligner cleaning solution called Steraligner. All I have to say is that it is amazing! It works so well. I now use it to clean my retainers.

- Invisalign aligners are not retainers. They are high-tech, removable braces. The thing is that they look a lot like retainers and they are removable like retainers. Thus, if you are an Invisalign patient, make sure you develop the habit of putting your aligners in your case when you take them out. And don't leave them just lying about. I promise that your dog can't tell the difference between a retainer and an Invisalign aligner. Furthermore, you can always count on Murphy's Law, and your dog will eat your aligner on a Saturday when your orthodontist's office is closed. I always tell my patients that wear retainers, "If it's not in your face, it's in the case!" You would do well to abide by this rule so that your aligners stay safe or do not get lost or accidentally thrown out.

- If you need to travel, remember to take your "braces" (aka aligners) with you if your travel dates coincide with your aligner change-out date. The last thing you want is to be in another state or country when you discover that today is the day you're supposed to change your aligners and you didn't bring the new ones with you. Only bring the ones you will need so that you don't risk losing the other ones.

- If you find that you're having trouble remembering to reinsert your aligners after eating, simply use your smartphone timer and set an alarm for yourself to remind you. It is easy to forget to put them back in, especially in the beginning or in a social setting. Having an alarm go off is a great way to help you remember.

As I've mentioned on multiple occasions, one of the huge benefits of wearing Invisalign or clear aligners is that it will be a lot quicker and even easier to clean your teeth.

- You may want to consider investing in an aligner removing tool. This is especially true if you don't have long finger nails to help you remove your aligners. The most popular one is called the "Outie Tool," and a six-pack can be purchase on Amazon for a little over $20.

- You can't chew gum with your aligners in. I tried. They will quickly stick to your aligners. If you are a habitual gum chewer and are considering Invisalign, this is something to think about.

Whether you choose fixed traditional braces or clear aligners, it is important to prepare yourself for some lifestyle changes. Therefore, it's good to know them ahead of time so you know what to expect. I firmly believe that lifestyle is an important consideration, so don't be shy about bringing up lifestyle questions at an orthodontic consultation.

Chapter 9

ORTHODONTICS IS A TEAM SPORT

"Alone we can do so little. Together we can do so much."
Helen Keller

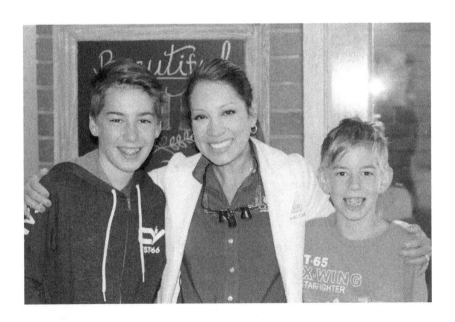

Like most great accomplishments in life, getting a beautiful smile is not something that is accomplished by one person only. It is in fact, a team sport. Think of your orthodontist as the team captain, with his or her clinical assistants as key players. Sounds great, right? Well did you know that you, the patient, are also one of the key players? That's right. We can't do this without you. And while we will do most of the work in creating your new smile, an important part of it depends on you (or your child). This is an important thing to consider before starting orthodontic treatment.

If we could follow you around everywhere to remind you what to do, we would probably do it. That's how much we care about your smile. The reality is that you have to want to do your part, and having us following you around is extremely creepy. So where does that leave us? If you want to have the best result possible from your or your child's orthodontic treatment, then the best thing to do is to follow your orthodontist's instructions.

Your orthodontist and their team are always there to help you and cheer you on.

The good news is that your part is easy. Furthermore, your orthodontist and their team are always there to help you and cheer you on. Let's explore your role in your smile journey a little more.

Good Oral Hygiene

The importance of maintaining good oral hygiene through brushing and flossing cannot be stressed enough. Plaque left behind on, or in between, teeth can lead to swollen, tender, and bleeding gums, white spots due to enamel calcium loss, and dental cavities. Additionally, braces that are covered in plaque are difficult to adjust and work around, so this can cause delays in your treatment.

Keeping your teeth clean with braces is easier than ever thanks to smaller brackets and other technological advances that allow orthodontists to treat your smile with minimally invasive appliances.

Really, the trick is knowing what you're doing, and this is where we can help you. Below are some simple tips:

- Consider investing in an electric toothbrush. Electric versus manual toothbrush has always been a topic for discussion, and while it is true that the most important thing is brushing technique, I strongly believe an electric toothbrush edges out the competition in the battle of the toothbrushes. Many dental studies support this as well.

- Brush gently at a forty-five-degree angle toward the gum line and around the top and bottom of the braces, moving the toothbrush in a small circular motion across all surfaces of the teeth in order to effectively remove plaque, as well as any trapped food particles.

- Brush at least three times per day, preferably after each meal, for a minimum of two minutes. Use a timer if needed.

- Replace your toothbrush or brush head every three to four months, or sooner if it shows signs of wear or if you have a cold or any other illness.

- Make it a point to look for clean and shiny braces, with the edge of the brackets clearly visible, as fuzzy or dull-looking metal can indicate poor brushing habits.

- Floss at least once per day to remove bacteria and any food that has accumulated, taking advantage of tools like floss threaders and Waterpiks if you are having difficulty getting into the tighter spaces.

- Use antimicrobial and fluoride mouthwashes, such as ACT mouth rinse.

By far, one of the best ortho-dontists in our area! The staff are all amazing and they treat you with much kindness and respect, the atmosphere at this place is very welcoming! I highly recommend people needing or wanting braces to choose this place.

—*Fidel G.*

- Use fluoride toothpaste and a toothbrush with soft, rounded bristles.

- Make the interdental brush part of your cleaning routine. As discussed in Chapter 8, an interdental brush is a small brush used to clean between the teeth and can be gently used to clean underneath and around your wires and braces where a regular toothbrush can't reach. It kind of looks like a mini bottle-cleaning brush or mini white Christmas tree and can be found at any drug store dental aisle or online stores like Amazon. Use an interdental brush to remove large pieces of debris before brushing with your normal toothbrush.

- Always use a mirror to check to make sure you haven't missed anything.

Wear Your Rubber Bands

Braces or aligners like Invisalign do a fabulous job of straightening your teeth. However, that doesn't mean your bite has been corrected. After all, you can have straight teeth on your top jaw and straight teeth on your bottom jaw, but that doesn't mean your teeth fit well together. That is, you can have straight teeth with an unhealthy bite. Furthermore, straight teeth alone will not give you the beautiful smile that you want.

Case in point: imagine someone with perfectly straight teeth on top and bottom but they have a large overbite that causes the lower lip to slide behind the upper teeth. Not the look you're after. The point is that correcting your bite is important and very often to correct your bite, you will need to wear rubber bands. Rubber bands are small elastics that you hook onto the braces of specific teeth. They usually come in a small bag of one hundred elastics. Rubber bands connect your upper teeth to your lower teeth in order to bring your teeth together in a specific way and thereby correct your bite.

Wearing your rubber bands the wrong way can actually worsen your bite, so if you have any doubts about how to wear them, don't be shy about asking questions until you are crystal clear.

There are many ways to wear your rubber bands, since how you wear them depends on the type of bite you have. The important thing is to follow your orthodontist's instructions faithfully so that you not only get the best result possible, but also get it in a timely manner, since not wearing your rubber bands can cause delays in your treatment. But never fear. Wearing your rubber bands can be challenging for the first few days but it is really easy once you get used to them. Below are some tips for successfully wearing your rubber bands:

- Make sure you understand how you're supposed to wear them. Wearing your rubber bands the wrong way can actually worsen your bite, so if you have any doubts about how to wear them, don't be shy about asking questions until you are crystal clear. If you are a parent and you see your child walking out of his or her appointment with rubber bands, be sure you also understand how your child should be wearing their rubber bands. One thing I always suggest to my patients is to take a "rubber band selfie" with their cell phone to help them remember how to wear their rubber bands. You can also ask for a diagram card to help you remember, but like most pieces of paper, this gets lost. A cell phone picture is your best bet.

- Make sure you understand how long to wear them. In general, rubber bands can be worn "full-time" or "night-time." In our office, full-time means twenty-four hours per day unless you are having a meal or cleaning your teeth. Night-time means eight hours per night while you sleep. If you wear your rubber bands at night-time but you were supposed to wear them full-time, you won't really get any correction.

- If it helps, ask for a second bag of elastics. When I was in braces, I had a bag in my car and a bag in my purse. If, for some reason, I forgot to put my rubber bands in my purse (this would sometimes happen when I switched purses), then I could get them from my car. For your teen, this could be a bag at home and one at their school locker. Point is, have a backup plan.

- If you or your child are wearing night-time rubber bands, set an alarm on your cell phone to help remind you that rubber bands must go on before going to bed.

- If you run out of rubber bands before your next appointment, don't say, "Yay! I get small break." Instead, stop by your orthodontist's office to pick up another bag. In our office, we will even mail them to you!

Rubber bands are "all or nothing." There are no moral victories in football or in rubber band wear. You either wear them 100 percent of the time (or close to it) or you don't. This is the most challenging concept for many of my young patients to understand. They think that if they wear their rubber bands 50 percent of the time, they will get 50 percent of the result. Unfortunately, there are no participation trophies in rubber band wear. This sounds tough, but I come from a place of love. Orthodontic tooth movement is the result of light continuous forces and 50 percent is not continuous. If your orthodontist asks you to wear rubber bands 24/7, take this as literally as possible. That way, you can be done with your rubber bands and your treatment as soon as possible.

If One of Your Braces or Attachments Comes Off, Let Your Orthodontist Know Right Away

Today's technology has allowed us to use smaller and smaller braces that stay bonded to your teeth with higher-than-ever bond strengths so that they stay put on your teeth throughout your entire treatment, despite their small size. That being said, nothing is indestructible. And there is a limit to the bond strength we can use to glue on your braces or else your enamel would be at risk of damage when your treatment is over and it is actually time to remove them on purpose. The best thing to prevent your braces or attachments from coming off is to avoid crunchy, hard, or sticky foods, as discussed in Chapter 8.

However, we understand that things happen, so if a bracket or attachment comes off, it is important that you call your orthodontic office right away. Depending on where you are in treatment, having a bracket or attachment off may cause delays in your treatment if not repaired right away. If it happens, don't just say, "I'll get it fixed when I go in in five weeks." Call the office and ask for guidance on what to do. In some cases, it is perfectly fine to wait, but by calling, you have advised your office so that they can either add more time to your next appointment to fix it or, if that's not possible, switch your appointment to a different time where enough time to fix your bracket is available. In other cases, especially when you are near the end of treatment, it is important that you go in as soon as possible to get the broken bracket repaired. Bottom line, if you have a bracket or attachment that has come off, call your office right away to avoid any potential delays in your treatment.

Doing Your Part Can Be Fun!

After reading all this, you may be thinking that getting orthodontic treatment is a lot of work. I can assure you that it is not. Especially when you have an awesome orthodontic team supporting you and cheering you on.

At Castilla Orthodontics, we have games and contests to support our patients through this journey and help them do their part. We have a quarterly hygiene contests that rewards patients (and their hygienist) for going to their dentist to get a professional cleaning. We also have a token program where patients can earn Castilla Ortho Tokens for doing a good job at cleaning their teeth or not having any broken brackets. These tokens can be saved up and then used to buy fun items at our office, such as gift cards, toys, and movie passes.

If you are searching for an orthodontist for your child, ask if the office you visit offers any fun incentive programs to help your child do their part as a Key Member of his or her orthodontic team.

Chapter 10

THE SMILE OF YOUR LIFE

"Every story has an end. But in life, every end is just a new beginning."
Dakota Fanning (*Uptown Girls*)

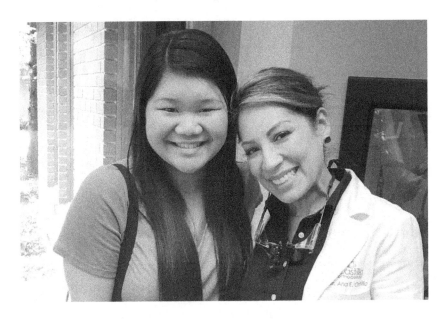

When you are done with your braces or Invisalign treatment, you will be as happy as anyone is at the end of a long journey. Finally, you have a beautiful smile. Let the compliments begin. I got my braces removed seventeen years ago and I get compliments on my smile almost every day. That being said, I don't think it's the smile itself. I think it's the confidence you have when you smile, knowing that your teeth look great, that attracts other people and results in compliments. That confidence is irresistible.

When your braces or attachments come off, it may seem like your journey toward a beautiful smile has ended, but the only thing that has ended is the "active" part of your treatment. That is, the part where your teeth are actively being moved by your orthodontic appliances. Now you enter the "retention" phase. And this phase is just as important as the active treatment phase because, believe me, when your braces come off, your teeth (with very rare exceptions) will want to move right back where they used to be.

So what does this retention phase look like? Well, every orthodontist treats this phase slightly differently. But, in general, it involves you getting, at the very least, a retainer for your upper teeth and a retainer for your lower teeth. A retainer is an appliance that holds your teeth in place so that they remain straight and aligned. The reason a retainer is needed is because, with very few exceptions, your teeth will start moving back the moment the braces are removed. This is difficult for a lot of people to believe or accept, but if you understand human anatomy and physiology, it makes perfect sense.

> *The reason a retainer is needed is because, with very few exceptions, your teeth will start moving back the moment the braces are removed.*

Teeth are not fused to your jaw bone. If they were, we wouldn't be able to move them. Instead, the roots of teeth are connected to the bone via elastic fibers called *periodontal ligaments*. These ligaments get stretched when the teeth are moved, and because they have some type of memory, the teeth will go back in the direction of their original positions when the braces or full-time aligners are no longer holding them in place. This is especially true if the patient started with severe rotations or spaces between their teeth. This is not to be looked at as a negative thing, but simply a fact of how our bodies works. Everything in our bodies is dynamic. Our skin changes over time, our eyesight changes over time. So do teeth.

In fact, even if you never get braces, your teeth will naturally become more crooked over time as your teeth age. This is a fact. So we go to the gym to keep up our bodies in shape, and we get facials to help keep up our skin, and we keep up with our eye appointments so we can see. By that same token, we need to wear retainers to keep our teeth straight. Think of it as part of your nightly routine.

There Are Different Types of Retainers

Like the braces themselves, retainers come in different forms, and it is up to you and your orthodontist to decide which one is best for you. Retainers are either removable or fixed, which means they cannot be removed and stay "fixed" on your teeth.

There are two main types of removable retainers, Hawley retainers and vacuum-formed retainers (often known as Essix or Clear retainers). Each type of retainer can be made for the upper or lower teeth. The Hawley retainers are made of an acrylic plate that covers the roof of the mouth on the upper and wraps around the tongue side of the teeth on the lower. This acrylic can be made of different colors or even patterns. Additionally, it has metal clasps that go over the back teeth and a metal wire that runs across the front teeth, holding them in place. This is a more traditional type of retainer and it has its advantages and disadvantages.

Dr. Castilla and her staff love on each of our children each time we walk through the door. They have been honest, fair, and competitive in pricing, while also having a top-of-the-line atmosphere that makes appointments fun for kids and their families, too!

—*Angie J.*

Vacuum-formed or clear retainers, on the other hand, are made of a clear plastic that wraps around all the visible surfaces of all your teeth. They look very, very similar to Invisalign or other aligners. Like Hawley retainers, clear, "Essix-type" retainers have their advantages and disadvantages. Most orthodontists have a preference of one retainer type over another, so this is something that is good to discuss with your orthodontist before starting treatment.

Additionally, you can also get fixed retainers. Fixed retainers consist of a wire that is glued behind your front teeth to keep them from moving. They are not often placed on the upper but when they are, the wire is glued to each and every front tooth. On the lower, the fixed retainer wire extends across all the front teeth and is glued to each and every front tooth or is glued only to the canines if a heavier wire is used.

Most orthodontists either use removable retainers only or a combination of removable and fixed retainers. I personally use a combination, since I strongly believe that most people will benefit from a fixed lower retainer, because the lower front teeth are the teeth that are most likely to relapse or move.

That being said, I do feel that the type of retainer that is chosen for a patient should be based on each patient's individual case. For example, most of my patients get clear retainers with a fixed retainer on the lower front teeth. However, I do make exceptions and will, on occasion, recommend a Hawley retainer to a patient. On other occasions, I will recommend a bonded retainer behind the upper two front teeth in addition to the removable retainer. I do this when someone starts out with gaps or spaces between their upper front teeth, since these types of spaces have a tendency to re-open otherwise.

Dental hygiene and home care should also be a consideration for retainer selection. While it is not difficult to floss around a fixed retainer once you learn how, removable-only retainers should be considered for any patients who have poor dental hygiene habits. As you can see, most patients will get the same type of retainer, but at the end of the day, it is still a case by case decision. As it should be.

Wear Your Retainers as Instructed

Once you have your retainers, it is extremely important that you wear them exactly as your orthodontist instructs. You have put a lot of time, energy, and money into your new smile. I'm sure you don't want your teeth to move. Often times, there is a short period during which you will need to wear your retainer twenty-four hours a day. This is quickly followed by switching the wear to night-time only (in your sleep), provided everything is going well and your teeth are staying put.

It is also important to come in for any retainer checkups that your orthodontist recommends, because this is how he or she checks that your retainers are working for you and that your teeth and bite are staying the way they are supposed to. Sometimes your orthodontist will need to make adjustments to how you wear your retainer based on what he or she is seeing.

Retainers for Life

Orthodontic retention is a lifelong commitment that is vital to keeping a beautiful and healthy smile. No retainer lasts forever. Therefore, at some point you will need to replace your retainer. At Castilla Orthodontics, we take this very seriously. We want your results to last, well, for life. This is, after all, the smile of your life. Not the smile of one year after braces. That is why we are proud to offer a Lifetime Retainer Program that makes it easier for our patients to obtain replacement retainers from our office. It is a retainer insurance, of sorts. When selecting an orthodontic office, you may want to ask about the cost of replacement retainers and understand the process for ordering replacement retainers in case you lose them or need to replace worn down ones.

Everyone always talks about retainer replacement due to wear and tear or loss, but one thing I never hear anyone discussing is the fact that retainers often have to be adjusted or replaced as a result of dental work. Dental work (especially crowns, veneers, and bridges) often changes the shape of your teeth. This would not be big deal except that your retainers were custom-made to fit your specific teeth. Thus, when you get any major dental work, it is common that your retainer won't fit afterward. If you get a filling, crown, bridge, or any other dental work, make sure to bring your retainers with you, so that your dentist can check that your retainer still fits after the dental work. In some cases, your dentist may be able to adjust the shape of your dental work to retroactively fit your retainer. In other cases, such as when you get veneers for peg lateral incisors or get a bridge, this will not be possible and you will have to go see your orthodontist for a new retainer.

When selecting an orthodontic office, you may want to ask about the cost of replacement retainers and understand the process for ordering replacement retainers in case you lose them or need to replace worn down ones.

Retainers Don't Keep Your Child from Growing

Oftentimes, when your child gets their braces removed, they are only thirteen or fourteen years old and their jaws and facial structures are still growing. This is especially true for boys who continue to grow much longer than girls. What does this mean? Fortunately, for the vast majority of children, the remaining growth is small and there is very little change to the bite.

However, there are a small number of children who get changes to their bite as a result of what's called "late mandibular growth," or continued growth of the lower jaw during adolescence. Most of the time, these changes are minor and will not require anything to be done. In other instances, the bite may change enough that retreatment may be considered. This is particularly true with the type of bite known as a Class 3 bite, where the patient either starts with an underbite or is close to having an underbite. The amount of growth that occurs after orthodontic treatment is complete is very difficult to predict and fortunately is not an issue for the vast majority of children. However, if your child starts out with an underbite or you are told he has a larger lower jaw, ask your orthodontist if extending the period of retention checks is advisable for your child.

This Is a Great Time to See Your Dentist

Once your braces or attachments come off, consider seeing your general dentist right away for a cleaning and exam with X-rays. Even though you should continue to see your dentist during your time in treatment, it is a lot easier to clean your teeth and look for cavities once your braces are out of the way. And of course, in order to keep your smile looking beautiful, you should continue to see your dentist regularly.

Whitening, Veneers and Other Cosmetic Services

One of the most common questions I get at the end of orthodontic treatment (especially from adult patients) is, "What's the best way to whiten my teeth?" or, "Do you offer whitening?" This is perfectly understandable. Your teeth are straight. Your smile is beautiful. Whitening can be the icing on the cake. When I got my braces off, the first thing I did pick up a box of Crest Whitening Strips to whiten my teeth. For that reason, our office gives some professional

The end of orthodontic treatment is a misnomer, as it is not so much an end as it is the beginning of your beautiful smile.

grade whitening gel to each adult patient as part of their Braces Off Gift, for them to use with their clear retainers. We also sell refill syringes and custom whitening trays for those who wish to get them. That being said, it's important to know when to whiten. If your braces have just come off, I recommend that you get a cleaning first as well as any cavities fixed before starting the whitening process.

Additionally, as I explained in Chapter 6, adult patients sometimes need to see their dentist to get composite bonding or veneers to restore or build up teeth that have been worn down by years of a bad bite. If this is you, the time to whiten your teeth is after your cleaning but before you get any cosmetic work done on your front teeth. This is because porcelain, composite resin, or any of the tooth-colored materials used to restore the look and shape of your front teeth cannot be whitened by dental whitening gel. Only natural tooth enamel can be whitened. Thus, you don't want to whiten after your veneers are done. They won't whiten. Instead, whiten your teeth first so that all the surrounding teeth are of a lighter shade. Then, when it is time to get your composite build-up or veneers, your dentist can match the porcelain or composite color to the shade of the newly whitened surrounding teeth.

A Beautiful Smile for Life

The end of orthodontic treatment is a misnomer, as it is not so much an end as it is the beginning of your beautiful smile. Like everything else in your body, your smile needs lifelong care and maintenance to keep it looking good. Wearing your retainers is just one small aspect. Visiting your dentist, eating a healthy diet, and good daily home care are also part of part of keeping your smile beautiful. For life.

Conclusion

A beautiful smile is so much more than just straight teeth. It is health, confidence, and joy. It is what you display during the happiest moments of your life. When you graduate from school, you smile. When you get married, you smile. When your child is born, you smile. It is, I dare say, a reflection of your spirit. And make no mistake, it can change your life. If nothing else, I hope I have conveyed that in this book.

The prospect of orthodontic treatment can seem daunting. Especially since there is so much seemingly conflicting information out there on the internet. I hope this book has provided you with the knowledge to feel confident that you too can find a great orthodontist and get a wonderful result from your treatment. Everyone deserves a beautiful smile and there is no reason you or your loved one cannot have one. So go out there and get the smile of your life.

Ana Castilla, DDS, MS
Diplomate, American Board of Orthodontics

Acknowledgments

Like just about anything else I do in my life, I could not have written this book without the loving patience and support of my husband, Eddy. Thank you for always believing in me and my dreams.